The DeFlame Diet

for

Immune Health

David R. Seaman, DC, MS

www.DeFlame.com
www.DrDavidSeaman.com

Find out how a pro-inflammatory diet and lifestyle puts you at greater risk when exposed to the coronavirus or flu virus

Shadow Panther Press

Wilmington, NC

Disclaimer

This book is intended as an educational volume only; not as a medical or treatment manual. The information contained herein is not intended to take the place of professional medical care; it is not to be used for diagnosing or treating disease; it is not intended to dictate what constitutes reasonable, appropriate or best care for any given health issue; nor is it intended to be used as a substitute for any treatment that may have been prescribed by your doctor. If you have questions regarding a medical condition, always seek the advice of your physician or other qualified health professional.

The reader assumes all responsibility and risk for the use of the information in this book. Under no circumstances shall the author be held liable for any damage resulting directly or indirectly from the information contained herein.

Reference to any products, services, internet links to third parties or other information by trade name, trademark, suppliers, or otherwise does not constitute or imply its endorsement, sponsorship, or recommendation by the author.

Cover design by: www.100covers.com

ISBN: 979-8663758987

Table of Contents

About Dr. David Seaman

Dr. Seaman has been studying the relationship between diet and chronic inflammation since 1987. In 2002, he wrote one of the first, if not the absolute first, scientific article that outlined the dietary induction of chronic inflammation:

> Seaman DR. The diet-induced proinflammatory state: a cause of chronic pain and other degenerative diseases? J Manipulative Physiol Ther. 2002;25:168-79.

He has written many other scientific papers that focus on pain, obesity, and chronic inflammation. His scientific papers have been cited by researchers at Harvard Medical School on three occasions, as well as by many researchers at other universities in America, Canada, Brazil, Europe, Russia, Middle East, Africa, India, China, and Australia.

You can follow Dr. Seaman at www.DeFlame.com and www.drdavidseaman.com, as well as at DeFlame Nutrition on YouTube and Facebook, and @DeFlameDoc on Twitter.

The DeFlame book series

The original DeFlame book entitled, *The DeFlame Diet: DeFlame your diet, body, and mind,* is about 250 pages long and discusses how a diet that is rich in refined sugar, flour, and oils leads to a state of chronic inflammation and then to the expression of chronic pain and disease. Specific diseases are not discussed in any detail because they all manifest as a consequence of the same underlying diet-induced pro-inflammatory state.

In the original DeFlame Diet book, I also discuss the anti-inflammatory benefits of whole foods and devote specific chapters to omega-3 fatty acids, potassium, magnesium, vitamin D, probiotics, saturated fats, trans fats, cholesterol, and many other topics. These topics are not discussed in detail in subsequent DeFlame books entitled, *The DeFlame Diet for Breast Health and Cancer Prevention* and *The DeFlame Diet to Stop Your Joints, Muscles, and Bones From Rotting.*

The purpose of these follow-up DeFlame books is to discuss how various conditions manifest as a consequence of living on pro-inflammatory foods. These books allow people to better understand their conditions and for whom a pro-inflammatory diet plays a causative role.

Amazon allows customers to look through the Table of Contents of each book, which allows a reader to identify if the book suits their needs. The original DeFlame Diet book has an introductory chapter about immune function, but does not remotely go into the detail that you will find in this current book.

Introduction

I was motivated to write *The DeFlame Diet for Immune Health* due to the novel coronavirus called SARS-CoV-2, which stands for "severe acute respiratory syndrome coronavirus 2." SARS-CoV-2 emerged from Wuhan, China at the end of 2019 and the ensuing pandemic and lockdown that occurred throughout the world in early 2020. COVID-19 (coronavirus disease of 2019) is the name of the disease that is caused by SARS-CoV-2. Coronaviruses derive their name from the fact that under electron microscopic examination, each virion is surrounded by a "corona," or halo.

At the time I began writing this book, I had already put up ten videos on my DeFlame Nutrition YouTube channel that addressed important issues to consider whenever the human body is challenged by an external stressor, for the purpose of becoming more resilient. The external stressor in question in these videos was of course SARS-CoV-2; however, the information generally applies equally to all challenging external stressors that humans are faced with, such as physical injury and psychological stressors. In other words, my YouTube videos and this book are not about "treating" viruses. They are about making the body more resilient to external threats, whether they be physical, psychological, bacterial, or viral. In this book, I will demonstrate that COVID-19 is actually a health crisis and NOT a virus crisis.

Consider that SARS-CoV-2, or any other virus that moves through the human population acting as an external threat, will affect people differently. Some will have no symptoms at all, which means these people are resilient. In contrast, others who are less resilient may feel like they have a cold; others will feel like they have mild flu symptoms; others feel like they have the worst flu of their life; others have such bad symptoms they go to the hospital; while others have such severe symptoms that they die in a hospital's ICU. It is important to understand that the same coronavirus was responsible for all of these varied responses. In other words, the SARS-CoV-2 was the same; however, the prevailing health and related resiliency of the bodies of the infected individuals were very different in order for such varied outcomes to manifest.

In the DeFlame world, we determine one's health status by tracking inflammatory markers. A truly healthy person will have normal inflammatory markers, so when they are exposed to an inflammation-stimulating agent like SARS-CoV-2, these people may have absolutely no symptoms or just mild symptoms that are bothersome for a few days. In contrast, as people become progressively more inflamed, they manifest more symptoms and more severe symptoms. Unfortunately, death can be the potential outcome for people who are highly inflamed.

Anyone who has watched the news about COVID-19 knows that people with pro-inflammatory pre-existing conditions, referred to as comorbidities, are at a much greater level of risk for complications when infected with SARS-CoV-2. These pro-inflammatory pre-existing conditions include diabetes, heart disease, chronic lung disease, moderate to severe asthma, severe obesity (BMI of 40 or greater), chronic kidney disease, and severe liver disease (1).

All of these conditions represent heightened states of inflammation. To verify this, you can do an internet search with "name of pro-inflammatory condition and inflammation" and you will see that dozens of scientific articles appear. In other words, if you search for "obesity and inflammation" you will see dozens of papers that explain how obesity is a state of chronic inflammation. The same holds true for all of the other pre-existing conditions cited by the CDC. This means that pre-existing inflammation is a health crisis and the real determinant of SARS-CoV-2 infection outcomes.

The purpose of this book is to demonstrate how a pro-inflammatory diet and lifestyle places you at a much greater risk for developing a severe outcome if you suffer from an infection. This requires that you learn about how the immune system functions in health and disease, which is dramatically altered when one becomes chronically inflamed.

References

1. CDC website. Article title: People who are at higher risk for severe illness. https://www.cdc.gov/coronavirus/2019-ncov/need-extra-precautions/people-at-higher-risk.html

Chapter 1
The human microbiome and virome
Basics you need to know

When we think of the human body, we mostly view it as consisting of skin, bones, muscles, a nervous system, and a bunch of organs (gut, heart, liver, kidneys, etc.). While this is true, at a microscopic level the human body is made up of trillions of human cells and a lot of water. The human body also contains trillions of non-human bacterial cells (the microbiome) and viruses (the virome), which outnumber human cells and perform essential functions that we need for survival.

Bacteria help digest our food, modulate immune function, protect us against other bacteria that cause disease, and produce vitamin K and some B vitamins, including vitamins B1, B2, and B12. There is approximately a 1:1 ratio of human and bacterial cells in our bodies (1). However, the human body's viral population outnumber bacteria. The largest population of viruses in our bodies are those that infect our bacteria, which are called bacteriophages. These bacteriophages modulate our bacterial population to support our symbiotic relationship with bacteria (2).

Healthy humans live in a symptom-free symbiotic relationship with their microbiome and virome. This relationship changes as we overeat refined food calories and become sedentary, which becomes especially obvious in the gut for most people, wherein the bacterial population grows beyond normal. This topic will be discussed in more detail in Chapter 12.

As stated above, the term microbiome refers to the bacterial population that lives on/in the human body. The first educational exposure to bacteria that I can remember was in a junior high school science class. We learned about various types of bacteria and had to identify them based on their structural characteristics. I even recall drawing different types of bacteria. In short, it is much easier for us to conceptualize bacteria in our microbiome than viruses in our virome.

The human virome is much more difficult to illustrate because viruses are so small and not taught in the visual fashion that we learn to recognize bacteria, so here are some revealing facts that should put the vastness of the human virome in context (2).

- A rough estimation based on bacteria-infecting viruses (bacteriophages) indicates that there are 100 times more viruses than human cells in the human body.
- Human-associated viruses control the microbial diversity of the human gut and skin.
- Our ancestral human-viral cohabitation is so profound that it is imprinted in our genome with approximately 100,000 known endogenous viral fragments, representing approximately 8% of our genome.

Multiple viruses, including coronaviruses and rhinoviruses (the viruses most associated with the common cold), are found in multiple body systems, including blood, nervous system, skin, respiratory tract, digestive tract, and genitourinary tract (2). This means that we are naturally inundated with and adapted to dealing with viruses – recall from above that 8% of our human genome is viral in nature. Based on this fact, it is difficult for me to conceptualize that a new virus, such as SARS-CoV-2, which causes the disease called COVID-19, would be a virus that our human physiology cannot manage.

Indeed, it turns out that in the younger population, unhealthy individuals who are typically obese and have high blood glucose levels are likely to develop the severe symptoms and complications of COVID-19 (3). In the elderly population, those who are frail and unwell are more likely to develop the severe cases of COVID-19 (3). In other words, as long as we are not too inflamed, our bodies can process SARS-CoV-2 without ill effect. This is why we have been told during the created crisis about COVID-19 that healthy people can be infected and have absolutely no symptoms. This also means that the clear message to the population should have been to get healthy, because when you are healthy, SARS-CoV-2 would be only a minor nuisance.

Strep throat may be the best example of how our symbiotic relationship with our microbiome changes and leads to a sore throat and related infectious symptoms. My perception is that a similar imbalance occurs with our virome. Consider that Streptococcus pyogenes (S pyogenes) is a bacterium that is part of the normal flora of our respiratory tract. S pyogenes is considered an opportunistic pathogen, which means that it will create an active infectious state, called strep throat, when we flame up our bodies.

Many pro-inflammatory stressors, outlined in Figure 1 on the next page, can flame us up and make us vulnerable to bacterial and viral infections. These are the same stressors that promote chronic pain, depression, heart disease, cancer, diabetes, Alzheimer's disease, and other chronic diseases.

Figure 1 illustrates the most common pro-inflammatory stressors that we all contend with to varying degrees. Each stressor causes our immune and other cells to release free radicals, prostaglandins, and cytokines, which are pro-inflammatory chemicals. Each chemical will be discussed in subsequent chapters, but for now you only need to understand that the over-production of these chemicals equates to a state of inflammation.

The only stressors that we cannot influence are our genetic makeup and the aging process, which is associated with an uptick of inflammation and is referred to as inflammaging in the scientific literature.

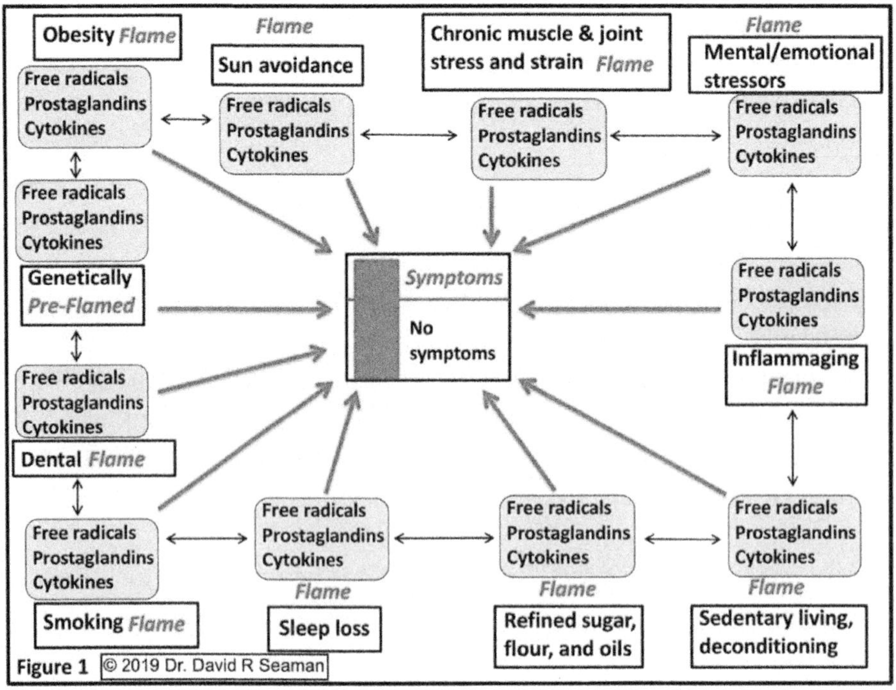

Figure 1 © 2019 Dr. David R Seaman

Notice that we can have an uptick of inflammation and as long as it stays below the threshold line, we can be symptom-free. Once we cross the line, symptoms develop, which means we all need to work on the various stressors to keep our level of inflammation at a normal level. Look at the various stressors and identify the ones you need to work on. The obvious focus of my books is the dietary flame, which is caused by an excessive consumption of refined sugar, flour, and oils.

In the context of COVID-19, it should be understood that we all are likely to be exposed to SARS-CoV-2; however, some people will have no symptoms and other people will develop COVID-19 symptoms and some may die from severe complications. The exact same virus can cause no symptoms, minor symptoms, severe symptoms, and even death. This tells us that the virus is NOT the problem…the problem is the prevailing health (inflammatory state) of the body that gets infected. In other words, the degree of body inflammation that we have when we are exposed to SARS-CoV-2 will determine where we will fall within the spectrum of possible symptoms. Chapter 4 outlines the various markers of inflammation that we can track to keep us in a DeFlamed state.

Infection science history you should know about

Louis Pasteur is credited for developing the "germ theory" of disease, which posits that pathogenic microbes invade the human body to cause disease. Pasteur was also involved in the initial development of vaccines. The term pasteurization is named after Pasteur and is achieved by heating milk and other foods to 212°F for the purpose of killing pathogens.

Almost everyone has heard of Pasteur. However, very few people have heard of his scientific rival named Antoine Bechamp, who is credited for developing what is called the "terrain theory" of disease. Bechamp argued that terrain (health of the body) was the determining factor for infectious diseases.

Based on the above information about Pasteur and Bechamp, it should be obvious that Bill Gates, Dr. Anthony Fauci, the media, and the government strongly embrace the germ theory. They believe that the power of SARS-CoV-2 can only be addressed by a vaccine. Interestingly, while Louis Pasteur was dying, he is alleged to have stated that, "Bechamp was right. The microbe is nothing. The terrain is everything."(4)

My personal view is that the both the germs and terrain (health of the body) must be taken into consideration. For example, if a DeFlamed healthy person drinks a glass of milk loaded with E Coli and Salmonella, they will likely get very, very sick. This means that both germs and body health need to be considered when determining the virulence of any bacteria or virus, especially when the government makes decisions that impact the entire population.

If you watched/read the news reports during 2020, you became aware of the term "comorbidities," which refers to one or more distinct conditions or diseases. The key comorbidities of concern for developing a severe case of COVID-19 are obesity, hypertension, and diabetes. In other words, we know that the health, or inflammatory status, of the terrain is the most significant factor that determines one's COVID-19 outcome. Despite this recognized fact, Gates, Fauci, the media, and the government are approaching COVID-19 as if the germ is everything and that the only way we can return society to normal is with a universal program of vaccination.

While I am not opposed to the judicious use of vaccines, it should be painfully obvious that Gates, Fauci, the media, and the government are all vaccine zealots. The have made absolutely no effort to encourage the population to become healthy, and therefore, resilient to SARS-CoV-2 and other future viruses that will likely emerge. This book will provide you with key health information that has been omitted from the public discourse revolving around COVID-19.

References

1. Sender R, Fuchs S, Milo R. Are we really vastly outnumbered? Revisiting the ratio of bacterial to host cells in humans. Cell. 2016;164:337-40.
2. Popgeorgiev N, Temmam S, Raoult D, Desnues C. Describing the silent human virome with an emphasis on giant viruses. Intervirology. 2013;56:395-412.
3. CDC website. Article title: People who are at higher risk for severe illness. https://www.cdc.gov/coronavirus/2019-ncov/need-extra-precautions/people-at-higher-risk.html
4. Zumla A, Maeurer M. Host-directed therapies for tackling multi-drug resistant tuberculosis: learning from the Pasteur-Bechamp debates. Clin Infect Dis. 2015;61:1432-38.

Chapter 2
COVID-19 vs the flu

As COVID-19 emerged, it was often compared to the seasonal flu for perspective. If level-headed scientists were invited to outline the details of this comparison, the similarities and differences could have been identified and clarified for the purpose of making sure that politicians, bureaucrats, the media, and the private sector had accurate knowledge about the nature of SARS-CoV-2. Unfortunately, this did not happen.

The key similarity between COVID-19 and the seasonal flu is that symptom severity is dependent on the prevailing health (inflammatory status) of the infected individual. In this context, both COVID-19 and the seasonal flu are essentially identical, which should be the message delivered to the general public in addition to emphasizing that the lung damage from SARS-CoV-2 appears to be more intense compared to a severe case of seasonal influenza.

Where COVID-19 and the flu differ the most is the manner in which SARS-CoV-2 gains access to and infects cells, especially lung cells that are called pneumocytes. This next sentence is likely to be a little confusing; however, to understand the COVID-19 infection process, we must discuss an important area of body chemistry. Scientists have identified that an area on the angiotensin converting enzyme-2 (ACE2) mediates the entry into the cell of three strains of coronavirus, those being SARS-CoV, NL63 and SARS-CoV-2 (1). ACE2 will make more sense to you by the time you finish reading this chapter.

While the ACE2 entry point for the coronavirus is the same for DeFlamed and inflamed people, the entry appears more aggressive in the flamed-up people. A key reason for this involves high blood glucose levels. For the average individual, the ultimate goal for a fasting glucose level is to be below 80 mg/dl. If you do not achieve this goal, you should at least get to 90 mg/dl or less. Once fasting blood glucose levels rise above 100 mg/dl, we now enter an abnormal prediabetic zone. Prediabetic individuals with fasting glucose levels between 100-125 mg/dl are typically classified as having the metabolic syndrome, which will be discussed more in Chapter 4. Fasting blood glucose levels above 125 mg/dl is considered to be in the type 2 diabetes zone.

One of the problems caused by high blood glucose levels, called hyperglycemia, is that it leads to a process called glycosylation, a scenario in which glucose excessively bonds to various body proteins. Anyone with the metabolic syndrome or diabetes should be aware of hemoglobin A1c, also called glycosylated hemoglobin, which essentially means "sugar-coated" hemoglobin. In other words, hyperglycemia leads to the "sugar-coating" of various body proteins, the most notable being hemoglobin in red blood cells. In normal individuals, less than 5.7% of hemoglobin is glycosylated, which means that a normal hemoglobin A1c level is below 5.7%. As A1c levels rise above 5.7%, this also means that there is an increase in the glycosylation of other body proteins, such as ACE2.

ACE2 is an enzyme that is characterized as a transmembrane protein and is found in lung cells, as well as in cells of the heart, blood vessels, gut, testes, brain, and kidney (1). Figure 1 illustrates that part of the enzyme is inside the cell, part of the enzyme traverses the cell membrane, and part of the enzyme exists outside the cell. The normal function of ACE2 is to convert circulating pro-inflammatory angiotensin II into anti-inflammatory angiotensin-(1-7). The relevance of this in terms of COVID-19 will be discussed shortly.

In addition to functioning as the angiotensin II converting enzyme, scientists discovered that coronaviruses could enter cells via ACE2. It turns out that glycosylated ("sugar-coated") ACE2 allows for a greater entry of SARS-Cov-2 into lung cells (2,3). You may have heard/read that people with type 2 diabetes are at a much greater risk for being compromised by COVID-19, and this is why.

Figure 1a illustrates the entry of SARS-CoV-2 into lung cells of DeFlamed people with normal glucose levels, compared to those with hyperglycemia (Figure 1b). The extra bold arrow in Figure 1b illustrates a greater lung cell entry by SARS-CoV-2 when ACE2 is glycosylated.

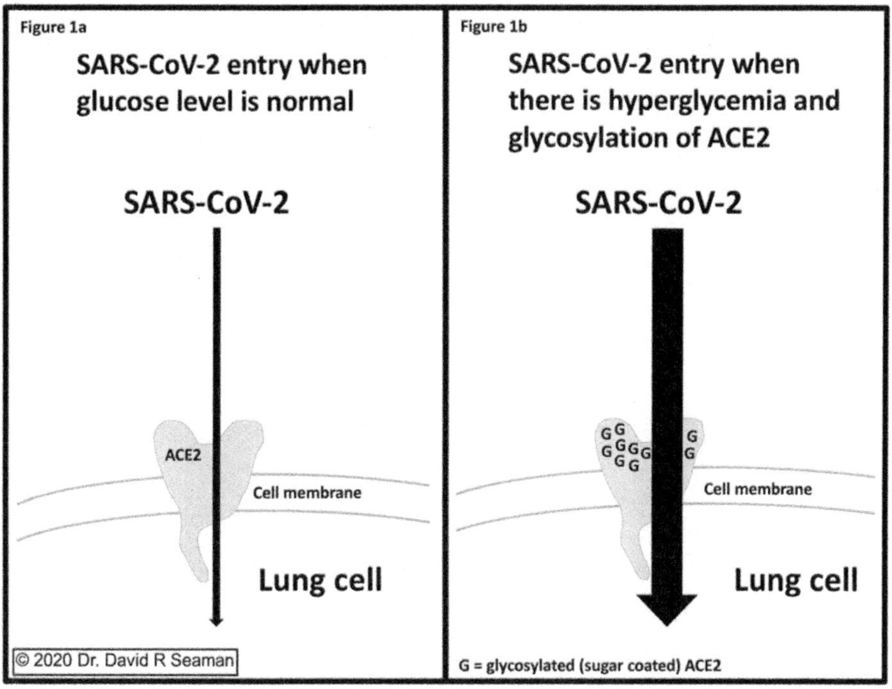

With Figure 1 in mind, it should be obvious why a key to preventing severe cases of COVID-19 is for people to get their blood glucose and A1c levels well into the normal range (2-4). This will prevent an excess of SARS-CoV-2 entry into lung cells and reduce COVID-19 symptom severity. It is shocking to me that a similar image was not created by the World Health Organization (WHO) and the scientists working with Dr. Fauci at the National Institutes of Health (NIH), for the purpose of imploring people to lose body fat and normalize their glucose levels.

There is another way in which ACE2 is involved in increasing the risk for developing a severe case of COVID-19. The ACE2 enzyme is part of a biochemical pathway in the human body called the renin-angiotensin system (RAS). The RAS is taught to healthcare practitioners in the context of blood pressure; however, there is so much more to the system that needs to be understood.

The key pro-inflammatory chemical in the RAS is called angiotensin II, which is a chemical that stimulates the nervous system to increase blood pressure. This is why two classes of drugs have been developed to address angiotensin II, which is overproduced in people with hypertension. One class of drugs is called angiotensin converting enzyme inhibitors (ACE inhibitors) and the other is angiotensin receptor blockers (ARBs). Table 1 lists the common brand names for each drug, which is followed by the generic name in parentheses.

Table 1

ACE inhibitors	**ARBs**
Accupril (quinapril)	Atacand (candesartan)
Aceon (perindopril)	Avapro (irbesartan)
Altace (ramipril)	Benicar (olmesartan)
Capoten (captopril)	Cozaar (losartan)
Lotensin (benazepril)	Diovan (valsartan)
Mavik (trandolapril)	Edarbi (azilsartan)
Monopril (fosinopril)	Micardis (telmisartan)
Prinivil, Zestril (lisinopril)	Teveten (eprosartan)
Univasc (moexipril)	
Vasotec (enalapril)	

While the common brand names of each class of drug would not alert us to the specific drug class, the generic names clearly indicate the class. Notice that all of the generic names of ACE inhibitors have a common suffix, that being "pril." In contrast, all generic names for ARBs have "sartan" as the common suffix.

Multiple millions of people take these classes of medications to treat high blood pressure, which is very important to appreciate because hypertension is a risk factor for developing a severe case of COVID-19, and this happens when someone has a pro-inflammatory angiotensin system. Figure 1 illustrates the various chemicals in the angiotensin chemical pathway. What you need to know is that angiotensin II is pro-inflammatory and can cause lung damage, while angiotensin-(1-7) is anti-inflammatory and prevents lung damage.

It is very important to understand that it is the prevailing inflammatory state of the body that determines if we produce a balanced amount of angiotensin II and angiotensin- (1-7). This means that we need to understand the lifestyle choices that lead us to a state wherein we create a pro-inflammatory angiotensin system…and this begins with the overproduction of angiotensinogen.

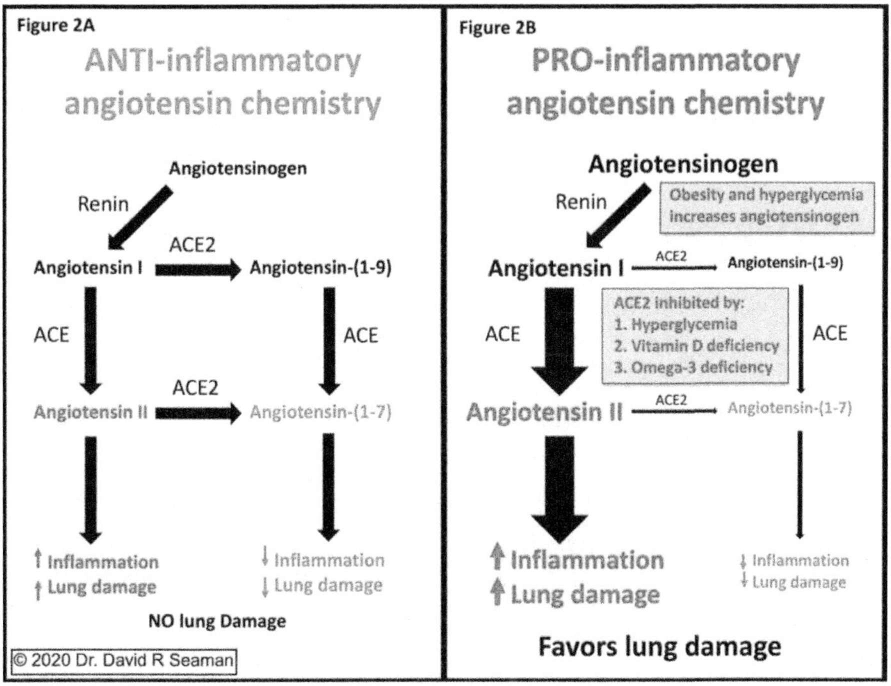

The liver is the primary source of angiotensinogen, which is overproduced when people have liver diseases, such as fatty liver (5,6), which develops due to the metabolic syndrome. Obese fat cells are also a source of extra angiotensinogen (7,8). This would probably be okay if the extra angiotensinogen was equally converted into angiotensin II and angiotensin- (1-7), however, this is not what happens. This is because the obese and hyperglycemic states inhibit the activity of ACE2 (1), which reduces the production of angiotensin- (1-7) and leads to its imbalance with angiotensin II that can promote lung damage as illustrated in Figure 2.

Figure 2A illustrates anti-inflammatory angiotensin chemistry found in non-obese individuals with normal blood glucose. Notice the balanced production of pro-inflammatory angiotensin II and anti-inflammatory angiotensin-(1-7), the outcome of which is no lung damage, and therefore, healthy lungs. Blood pressure will also be normal because blood pressure-elevating angiotensin II is not overproduced and is balanced by angiotensin-(1-7).

In contrast, Figure 2B illustrates pro-inflammatory angiotensin chemistry, wherein there is an overproduction of lung-damaging angiotensin II and a reduced production of lung-protecting angiotensin- (1-7), as indicated by larger font and arrow sizes. We also know that ACE2 activity is compromised when people lack adequate vitamin D and omega-3 fatty acids (9,10), which will also reduce the production of anti-inflammatory angiotensin- (1-7).

Because the human body is very resilient, people who are obese, hyperglycemic, and deficient in key nutrients like vitamin D and omega-3 fatty acids, are often able to manage okay for a while with a pro-inflammatory angiotensin system due to various medications for blood pressure and blood sugar. However, it should be understood that these people are still compromised. They live in a chronic pro-inflammatory state that favors lung damage and the development of chronic diseases, such as heart disease, cancer, Alzheimer's disease and others. All that is needed for lung damage to develop in these people is the right pro-inflammatory stimulus, such as SARS-CoV-2 infection.

Figure 3 illustrates what happens when a person with a pro-inflammatory angiotensin system is infected with SARS-CoV-2. Notice that SARS-CoV-2 infection further reduces the activity of ACE2, which means even less angiotensin-(1-7) production and a greater production of angiotensin II (1).

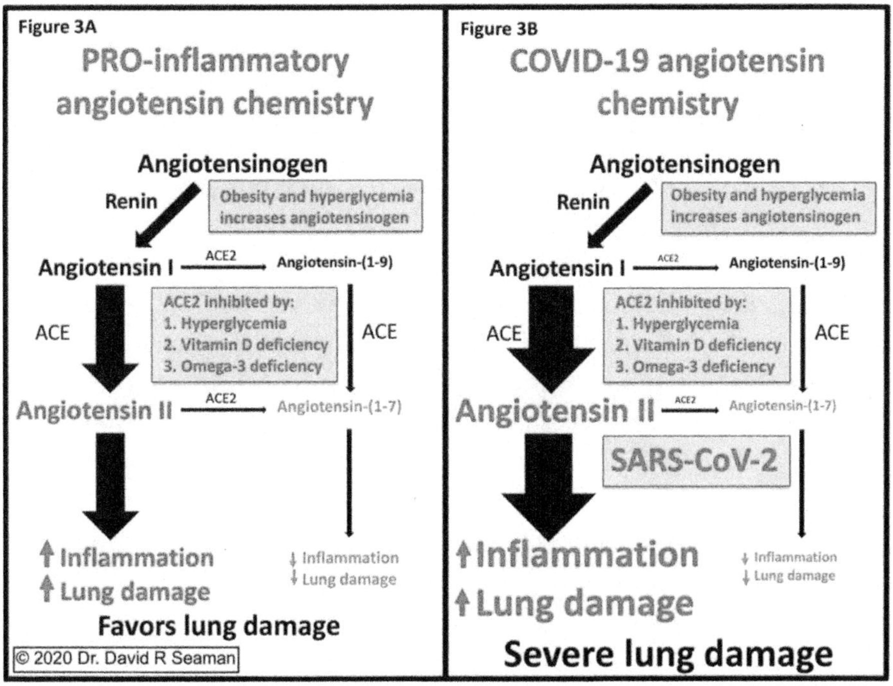

After reading this chapter, you should now be able to understand why it is that people who are obese, hypertense, and hyperglycemic are most likely the people who will have severe lung complications and may die from a SARS-CoV-2 infection. These same people are the ones who are far more likely to spread the virus to others. Indeed, obese hyperglycemic flamers stay infected longer, shed more viruses, and are far more contagious compared to the healthy asymptomatic individuals that have been blamed for spreading the virus (4).

In addition to what is described above, you should be aware of one more fact about angiotensin II, which is characterized as a pro-inflammatory chemical (11). Scientists have demonstrated that immune cells are activated by angiotensin II (1,12), which causes them to release pro-inflammatory cytokines and other inflammatory chemicals to heighten the inflammatory state that damages the body, whether one has COVID-19 or not. However, with SARS-CoV-2 infection, this is amplified because SARS-CoV-2 enters cells via

ACE2, which further amplifies the production of both angiotensin II and cytokines, which can promote a hyperinflammatory response called the cytokine storm (13). The cytokine storm is when cytokine production becomes especially excessive, which can cause certain people to die when they are infected by the coronavirus, flu virus, and other viruses (14,15).

A final point to consider is that this chapter focused on how SARS-CoV-2 and other coronaviruses enter lung cells to promote lung damage in those who are pre-flamed by obesity and hyperglycemia. The next dangerous virus that comes along may not be a coronavirus and will enter cells differently and could put other organs at risk of severe damage. This should not be your concern because no matter the virus and how it behaves, the key to getting through the infection process is to be DeFlamed. So your focus now and in the future should be to become as DeFlamed as you can, which means you should get all of the inflammatory markers (Chapter 4) into the normal range.

References

1. Verdecchia P, Cavallini C, Sapnevellow A, Angeli F. The pivotal link between ACE2 deficiency and SARS-CoV-2 infection. Eur J Intern Med. April 20, 2020 [Epub ahead of print].
2. Ceriello A. Hyperglycemia and the worse prognosis of COVID-19. Why a fast glucose control should be mandatory. Diabetes Res Clin Pract. 2020;163:108186.
3. Brufsky A. Hyperglycemia, hydroxychloroquie, and the COVID-19 pandemic. J Med Virol. 2020;92:770-75.
4. Luzi L, Radaelli MG. Influenza and obesity: its odd relationship and the lessons for COVID-19 pandemic. Acta Diabetologica. 2020;57:759-64.
5. Silva AC, Miranda AS, Rocha NP, Teixeira AL. Renin angiotenssin system in liver diseases: friend or foe? World J Gastroenterol. 2017;23:3396-406.
6. Wei Y, Clark SE, Thyfault JP et al. Oxidative stress-mediated mitochondrial dysfunction contributes to angiotensin II-induced nonalcoholic fatty liver disease in transgenic Ren2 rats. Am J Pathol. 2009;174:1329-37.
7. Harte A, McTernan P, Chetty R, et al. Insulin-mediated upregulation of the renin angiotensin system in human subcutaneous adipocytes is reduced by rosiglitazone. Circulation. 2005;111:1954-61.
8. Yanai H, Tomono Y, Ito K, et al. The underlying mechanisms for development of hypertension in the metabolic syndrome. Nutr J. 2008;7:10.

9. Ilie PC, Stefanescu S, Smith L. The role of vitamin D in the prevention of coronavirus disease 2019 infection and mortality. Aging Clin Exper Res. 2020; May 6:1-4.
10. Ulu A, Harris TR, Morisseau C, et al. Anti-inflammatory effects of omega-3 polyunsaturated fatty acids and soluble epoxide hydrolase inhibitors in angiotensin-II dependent hypertension. J Cardiovas Pharmacol. 2013;62:285-97.
11. Phillips MI, Kagiyama S. Angiotensin II as a pro-inflammatory mediator. Curr Opin Investig Drugs. 2002;3:569-77.
12. Benigni A, Cassis P, Remuzzi G. Angiotensin II revisted: new roles in inflammation, immunology and aging. EMBO Mol Med. 2010;2:247-57.
13. Mahmudpour M, Roosbeh J, Keshavarz M, et al. COVID-19 cytokine storm: the anger of inflammation. Cytokine. 2020;133:155151.
14. Liu Q, Zhou Y, Yang Z. The cytokine storm of severe influenza and development of immunomodulatory therapy. Cell Mol Immunol. 2016;13:3-10.
15. Tisoncik JR, Korth MJ, Simmons CP, et al. Into the eye of the cytokine storm. Microbiol Mol Biol Rev. 2012;76:16-32.

Chapter 3
How to prepare for a viral pandemic event

As far as I can tell, the governmental authorities that have the power to shut down the economy as they have done, have substantially overestimated the severity of the novel coronavirus (SARS-CoV-2) during the beginning of 2020. The powers that be, which are often referred to as "the powers that shouldn't be," have treated the coronavirus as if it has the same lethality as a Hollywood movie virus.

Multiple movies about killer viruses have been made and their lethality is drastically more severe compared to SARS-CoV-2, which causes COVID-19 that manifests as fever, dry coughing, and shortness of breath, from which most people recover. Only in the movies have we seen viral infections with the lethality to kill everyone who is infected unless an antiserum is rapidly developed.

In real life, no one has ever seen an infectious event that reached the extreme we saw in the movies *Outbreak* (1995) and *Contagion* (2011). For example, in *Outbreak*, which starred Dustin Hoffman and Renee Russo, both actors play CDC scientists who go into a town that became the epicenter of the fictional Motaba virus infection that was brought to America by a smuggled monkey.

Russo's character gets infected and within a day or two, she is almost dead – it is important to understand that anyone infected by a Hollywood movie virus tends to die in a gruesome fashion, which can subconsciously plant such images in our minds, which is what I think has happened to a large degree in relation to COVID-19. This is because, according to Business Insider, *Outbreak* was one of Netflix's most popular movies that people watched while locked down at home due to COVID-19 (1). Consider what this can mean for many people. They watch a scary virus movie wherein Motaba kills people within a few days. Then in real life, they are constantly bombarded by scary information about COVID-19, which allows for the subconscious mind and emotional brain to equate the SARS-CoV-2 coronavirus with Motaba in *Outbreak*. However, SARS-CoV-2 is a shockingly weak virus compared to Motaba.

Unlike a Hollywood movie virus like Motaba that kills anyone who gets infected, the 2020 coronavirus can have virtually no effect at all in people who are healthy. This means that COVID-19 is actually NOT a virus crisis; it is a health crisis. We know this to be the case because amidst the COVID-19 hysteria, we have also been told that infected healthy people often show absolutely NO SIGNS of being infected. So, the key message should LOUDLY urge unhealthy people to get healthy for the benefit of themselves, their families, and society at large.

To be clear, if we were all healthy and fit, very, very few of us would develop symptoms severe enough to require hospitalization and virtually no one would die, except for old frail people who are living in nursing homes and already close to death, which is the reason why most people live in nursing homes. Both of my grandmothers lived into their 90s and my great aunt lived to be 100. All three spent their remaining time in nursing homes, so I am very aware of the level of ill health that exists in nursing homes. I visited all three of them in their respective nursing homes, and based on that experience, I am amazed that some of these people are actually alive and it is quite obvious to me why an acute viral infection of any kind could be the final straw.

The best way to prepare for a novel virus like SARS-CoV-2, which causes COVID-19, is for the population to be healthy prior to becoming infected, so that the virus can silently sweep through society without ill effect for 99% of the people. Unfortunately, the American population is not remotely healthy. Americans are an extremely unhealthy and sick population. Over 70% of the US population is overweight or obese, and obesity is known to be a risk factor for having a severe reaction and complications when infected with a virus, which has been known by scientists for many years. So, take Bill Gates for example. He has done Ted Talks and television interviews about being concerned about the next pandemic virus...but he NEVER ever mentions that we should prepare by getting healthy so the American population is not unduly encumbered. Instead, Gates spends most of his time talking about vaccines.

In fact, we have been told by Bill Gates (who has zero medical training), Justin Trudeau (the Prime Minister of Canada with zero medical training), and Dr. Anthony Fauci (a bureaucrat "scientist"), that life will NOT return to normal until we are ALL vaccinated. Of additional interest to me is that many average Joes on the street, who also have no medical training, are following suit and claiming that we cannot resume our normal lives unless we all get vaccinated. The flu vaccine is an example how this unilateral approach is shortsighted.

If you go to the CDC website, it explains that people can still get the flu even if they were vaccinated because the flu vaccine can vary in how well it works in different people (2). Therefore, it is clearly foolish to think that our modern world cannot go back to normal, as Gates and others claim, until we all get vaccinated. To be clear:

> Did Bill Gates ever implore us to get healthy? **NO**
> Did Dr. Fauci ever implore Americans to get healthy? **NO**
> Did politicians tell Americans to get healthy while locked down? **NO**
> Did news channels spend time imploring Americans to get healthy? **NO**
> How many democrats in congress implored us to get healthy? **NONE**
> How many republicans in congress implored us to get healthy? **NONE**

Oddly enough, a so-called far left-wing political commentator named Van Jones urged his fellow black Americans to get healthy because a significant percentage are obese, diabetic, and hypertense, and therefore at a much greater risk for suffering from a potentially catastrophic outcome if infected by the coronavirus (3). Jones did not make this suggestion in an accusatory fashion; rather, he explained that he is someone who COVID-19 could kill, because he is in his early 50s and has high blood pressure, high cholesterol, and high blood sugar.

What Jones said is true for all people regardless of skin color or race. However, Jones presents himself as a voice for black America, which is why he directed his recommendation to his audience. As timing would have it, Jones' comments appeared at the same time an article was written in the *The Baltimore Sun*, which explained that 53% of COVID-19 deaths occurred from within the African American population, while 38% were white and 5.5% were Asian (4). This is especially concerning, as Maryland's black population at 30% is half the white population at 60% (4), which demonstrates how lethal COVID-19 has been for our black population. Instead of being thanked, Van Jones was slammed by some black people for promoting racism for singling out Black America to get healthy (3).

A similarly odd response occurred when, on May 5, 2020, singer-songwriter Adele posted a picture of herself on Instagram that revealed her 100-pound weight loss. She was properly complimented by some; however, others criticized her for fat shaming. According to an article in the British media outlet *Independent*, celebrating Adele's weight loss is not a compliment; rather, it is fatphobia.

I am not a participant in pop culture or identity politics so I do not understand how people can construe a person's choice to achieve a healthy body weight as fat shaming or being fatphobic or promoting racism. The new lean Adele is no longer at risk for developing diabetes and other conditions related to obesity, which means she is far less likely to develop complications if infected by SARS-CoV-2. In fact, Adele should be the poster woman for how to emerge from the coronavirus lockdown...lean, healthier, and much more resilient to physical, mental, and viral stressors.

With the above mind, all of America needs to get healthy and achieve a proper body weight and proper blood sugar regulation. However, you can see the dilemma we are in. No one in the public eye is robustly sounding the alarm that fat, sick people need to lose weight and get healthy so they do not die from the coronavirus, flu virus, or the next novel virus that emerges. And the one guy who does (Van Jones), gets accused of promoting racism by some of his fellow black Americans. In short, as far as I can tell, America will be terribly unprepared for the next pandemic scare as the health of America will continue to decline.

I personally do not care what color your skin is…be it black, brown, white, yellow, green or purple…everyone needs to DeFlame themselves back into a state of health so they can be more resilient to any challenging stressor, such as the novel coronavirus called SARS-CoV-2 that has compromised America and most other nations on earth.

As stated earlier in this chapter, COVID-19 should not be viewed as a virus crisis. It should be viewed as a health crisis. More specifically, this health crisis is a chronic inflammation crisis that is created by a pro-inflammatory immune system in response to our pro-inflammatory lifestyle.

References

1. https://www.businessinsider.com/coronavirus-outbreak-one-of-netflixs-most-popular-movies-2020-3
2. CDC website. Vaccine effectiveness: how well do the flu vaccines work? https://www.cdc.gov/flu/vaccines-work/vaccineeffect.htm
3. Jones V. I'm someone Covid-19 could easily kill. Here is what I am doing about it. CNN Opinion. Friday, April 24, 2020. https://www.cnn.com/2020/04/24/opinions/creating-a-pandemic-resistant-black-community-jones/index.html
4. Cohn M, Ruiz N, Wood P. Black Marylanders make up largest group of coronavirus cases as state releases racial breakdown for first time. Baltimore Sun. April 9, 2020.

Chapter 4
The DeFlame Diet basics

After discussing the reasons for why it is so important to become healthier, it is time to share how to do that. Table 1 outlines pro-inflammatory calories that should not be considered food and this is because real food contains nutrients, while pro-inflammatory calories lack nutrients or have nutrient imbalances. Table 1 also contains whole foods that constitute options for The DeFlame Diet. This table was first published in *The DeFlame Diet: DeFlame Your Diet, Body, and Mind,* which is the original DeFlame Diet book that contains 250 pages about the relationship between diet and inflammation. If you want the details about how whole foods and various key nutrients reduce body inflammation, then you should also read *The DeFlame Diet: DeFlame Your Diet, Body and Mind.*

Table 1 - Pro-inflammatory vs. DeFlame Diet vs. DeFlame Ketogenic Diet

Pro-inflammatory calories	**DeFlame Diet**	**DeFlame Ketogenic Diet**
Refined sugar	Grass-fed meat and wild game	Grass-fed meat and wild game
Refined grains	Meats	Meats
Grain flour products	Wild caught fish	Wild caught fish
Trans fats	Shellfish	Shellfish
Omega-6 seed oils (corn, safflower, sunflower, peanut, etc.)	Chicken	Chicken
	Omega-3 eggs	Omega-3 eggs
	Cheese	Cheese
	Vegetables	Vegetables
	Salads (leafy vegetables)	Salads (leafy vegetables)
	Fruit	** No fruit*
	Roots/tubers (potato, yams, sweet potato)	** No roots/tubers*
	Nuts (raw or dry roasted)	Nuts (raw or dry roasted)
	Omega-3 seeds: hemp, chia, flax seeds	Omega-3 seeds: hemp, chia, flax seeds
	Dark chocolate	** Sugar free dark chocolate*
	Spices of all kinds	Spices of all kinds

	Olive oil, coconut oil, butter, cream, avocado, bacon	Olive oil, coconut oil, butter, cream, avocado, bacon
	Red wine and dark beer	Red wine
	Coffee and tea (green tea is best option)	Coffee and tea (green tea is best option)
		* *No legumes and whole grains*

This current book about immune health will focus on how the pro-inflammatory calories "flame-up" the immune system and lead to poorer outcomes when one is exposed to an infectious agent. This is very important to understand as almost 60% of the average American's diet comes from these pro-inflammatory calories, which are implicated in the expression of all chronic diseases, including the severity of viral infections. This fact was even emphasized in an article in the New York Post (4/18/2020) entitled "*America's junk food diet makes us even more vulnerable to coronavirus.*"

When people find out about the disease-promoting nature of pro-inflammatory calories, they often react in a fashion that surprises me…they often first want to know the precise amount of junk food they are allowed to still eat to achieve good health. Fortunately, the guiding principle behind The DeFlame Diet addresses this issue, so it need not be a source of personal emotional turmoil.

The purpose of The DeFlame Diet is to normalize various markers of inflammation. It is that simple. Fortunately, we can achieve normal marker levels as vegans, omnivores, and even carnivores, so there are many diet options that are acceptable. My personal preference is to be an omnivore, with my first goal in mind being to avoid developing the pro-inflammatory metabolic syndrome outlined in Table 2.

Table 2 - Metabolic syndrome markers

Metabolic syndrome	Abnormal value	Date	Date	Date	Date
1. Fasting blood glucose	≥ 100 mg/dL				
2. Fasting triglycerides	≥ 150 mg/dL				
3. Fasting HDL	< 50 for women; < 40				

cholesterol	men				
4. Blood pressure	≥ 130/85				
5. Waist circumference	> 35″ women; > 40″ men				

An individual is considered to have the metabolic syndrome when at least 3 of the 5 markers in Table 2 are present. Almost 25% of adults between the ages of 40-49 have hyperglycemia (metabolic syndrome) and this rises to over 40% of adults age 60 and older (1), so it is a pervasive problem. It should be obvious that most of these metabolic syndrome markers become abnormal as we gain fat mass. Accordingly, the first biochemical need that applies to EVERYONE is a proper caloric balance. Overeating is the key problem to avoid.

No matter if one eats a vegan, omnivore, carnivore, Paleo, or ketogenic diet, calories can be over-consumed, which means that all of these diets can be pro-inflammatory. Conversely, if the caloric balance is proper, all of these diets can be anti-inflammatory. This is an especially important concept to understand, as overeating calories leads to obesity and the metabolic syndrome, which are known to increase the severity of a viral infection.

The challenge people have with giving up pro-inflammatory calories is that they taste really good and we crave them, which is why I use the term "dietary crack" to describe so-called "foods" made from sugar, flour, salt, and omega-6 oils. Breads, cakes, desserts, pretzels, donuts, French fries (and other deep-fried foods), cereals, etc., are the most notable caloric culprits to be avoided.

The easiest way to DeFlame your diet is to replace these calories with vegetation, which rapidly leads to a normalization of all inflammatory markers. If you are especially tempted by pro-inflammatory calories, I would recommend reading my book entitled, *Weight Loss Secrets You Need To Know,* which contains a host of mental strategies and information about how to avoid pro-inflammatory calories.

With the above information in mind, it should be understood that it is the cumulative effect of an excess consumption of pro-inflammatory dietary calories that is the key issue. In other words, eating a cookie every day at 100-200 calories would be irrelevant for the average person if all other pro-inflammatory factors in the diet were eliminated. Table 3 outlines multiple simple-to-measure inflammatory markers that we need to normalize. For the details about the various markers listed in Tables 2 and 3, they are discussed in *The DeFlame Diet* book.

Table 3 - General markers of inflammation

Pro-inflammatory markers	Parameters	Date	Date	Date	Date
Fasting glucose	65-80 mg/dl = ketogenic diet 80-90 = low carbohydrate diet < 100 = considered normal 100-125 = pre-diabetes >125 = type 2 diabetes				
2-hour postprandial glucose	<140 mg/dl = normal 140-199 = pre-diabetes 200+ = diabetes				
Hemoglobin A1c (HbA1c)	<5.7% = normal 5.7-6.4% = pre-diabetes ≥6.5% = type 2 diabetes				
Fasting triglycerides	<90 mg/dl predicts controlled postprandial response				
Fasting triglyceride/HDL ratio	>3.5 = oxidation of LDL cholesterol				
Blood pressure goal	Less than 120/80 = normal 120-139/80-89 = pre-hypertension 140-159/90-99 = Stage 1 hypertension ≥160/100 = Stage 2 hypertension				

Waist circumference goal - men	33″ or less				
Waist circumference goal - women	28″ or less				
Women waist/hip ratio (risk factor for type 2 diabetes = inflammation)	<0.80 = normal 0.81-.85 = moderate inflammation >0.85 = high inflammation				
Men waist/hip ratio (risk factor for type 2 diabetes = inflammation)	<0.95 = normal 0.96-1.0 = moderate inflammation >1.0 = high inflammation				
Body mass index (BMI)	18.5-24.9 = normal 25-29.9 = overweight ≥30 = obese				
hsCRP in mg/L (general marker of chronic inflammation)	<1.0 = normal 1.0-3.0 = mild/moderate inflammation >3.0 = high inflammation				
25(OH)D (vitamin D)	32-100 ng/ml (goal at least 60-80ng)				

The information presented thus far in this chapter represents the essence of The DeFlame Diet approach. Table 1 lists the pro-inflammatory calories that you should avoid, and also lists the whole foods that make up The Deflame Diet and The DeFlame Ketogenic Diet. The next step is to get your markers into the normal range. You can track several markers on your own at home, including fasting and postprandial glucose (with a glucometer), blood pressure, waist circumference, waist/hip ratio, and body mass index (BMI). For the lab tests, you will need to consult with a physician. By keeping track of the various markers, you will gain a sense of control over your health that you did not have before.

Regarding body weight, BMI, and waist/hip ratio, there is a slippery slope to avoid at all costs that needs to be understood. People can maintain these markers in the normal range on a diet of just French fries and donuts. In fact, you can be 100 pounds overweight and go on a 1000 calorie per day diet of just French fries and donuts and achieve a normal body weight. In this extreme case, you would achieve or maintain a normal body weight; however, you would be inflamed by an excess of omega-6 fatty acids from the oils used to make the French fries and donuts, as well as a lack of omega-3 fatty acids, magnesium, polyphenols/carotenoids, and other vitamins and minerals. The goal, as stated above, is to replace pro-inflammatory refined sugar, flour, and oil calories with vegetation.

How to measure waist/hip ratio and BMI

Waist circumference is measured at the umbilicus (belly button), which typically reflects the greatest area of abdominal girth, and thus, the presence or absence of abdominal obesity. For some people, the greatest abdominal girth is an inch above or an inch below the umbilicus. You want to measure where you have the most abdominal girth. You then divide the waist circumference by hip circumference.

The hip measurement should be done in a fashion to capture the most mass of the buttocks, which you typically find at the level of the greater trochanter. You find the greater trochanter at the top of the thigh bone. The greater trochanter is large and sticks out, so it is easy to feel. Put your hands on your buttocks, then slide them to the side and you will feel the greater trochanter of the thigh bone. Measure your hip circumference where you feel the greater trochanter.

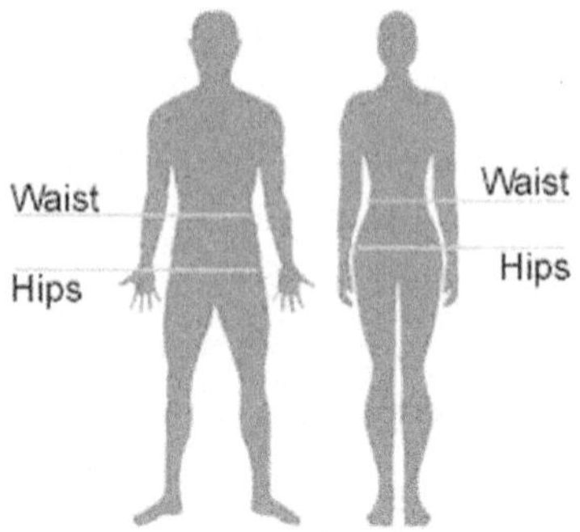

A normal waist/hip ratio for women is .8, which indicates that the waist measure should be less than the hip measurement. Anything higher than .8 reflects a gradual increase in ongoing inflammation.

A normal waist/hip ratio for men is .95, which again, indicates that the waist measure should be less than the hip measurement. Anything higher than .95 reflects a gradual increase in ongoing inflammation.

For BMI, you can do an internet search for BMI NIH, which will bring you to an NIH (National Institutes of Health) website that allows you to plug in your height and weight and then calculates your BMI. The utility of knowing your waist/hip ratio and BMI is that they typically correlate very well to the blood test markers of inflammation listed in Table 3. As values for waist/hip ratio and BMI rise, so do the blood test markers.

Time-restricted feeding

Fasting has become a popular topic in recent years and consequently, research has shown that fasting is anti-inflammatory. The challenge is choosing the best approach to take. My preference is called time-restricted feeding (TRF) because it is less stressful and challenging for most people compared to doing a water fast.

I think it is wise for everyone to fast at least 13 hours per night and try to extend it up to 18 hours based on one's individual comfort level, and this is because TRF is anti-inflammatory (2-4). Even if one eats pro-inflammatory calories, it is much better to do it in a 6-11 hour eating window. Consider this real-life example.

I met a guy who told me that at the age 45 he was diagnosed with type 2 diabetes. At the time of the diagnosis his weight was 250 pounds, while his proper weight was 200 pounds. Because he did not want to take medications for the rest of his life, this man decided to eat just 600 calories per day within a 6-hr time period until he got his weight back to 200 lbs. For 3 months he ate a double cheeseburger from MacDonald's, which was about 450 calories. The remaining 150 calories were from vegetables and fruit. At the end of the 3 months, he weighed 200 pounds again and no longer had diabetes.

I am not suggesting that anyone should do the double cheeseburger plan. The point of this example is to illustrate that there are many ways to DeFlame. My suggestion is to drastically avoid refined sugar, flour, and oils whether one chooses to be a vegan, omnivore, or carnivore and then let the normalization of inflammatory markers be the ultimate eating guide. In most cases, it is not a requirement for the diet to be ketogenic, which has become very popular in recent years. So only do a ketogenic diet if it suits your individual preferences and needs. Whichever foods you choose to eat, begin with a 13-hr fast and then extend it based on your comfort level, which can vary day to day.

In the context of a viral infection, especially with COVID-19 in mind, you can imagine how well this 45-year old guy reduced his chances of having complications if he happened to get infected. Both obesity and diabetes are risk factors for complications and even death.

References

1. Ford ES, Giles WH, Dietz WH. Prevalence of the metabolic syndrome among US adults: findings from the Third National Health and Nutrition Examination Survey. JAMA 2002;287:356–59.
2. Marinack CR, Nelson SH, Breen CI, et al. Prolonged nightly fasting and breast cancer prognosis. JAMA Oncol. 2016;2:1049-55.
3. Moro T, Tinsley G, Bianco A, et al. Effects of eight weeks of time-restricted feeding (16/8) on basal metabolism, maximal strength, body composition, inflammation, and cardiovascular risk factors in resistance-trained males. J Translational Med. 2016;14:290.
4. Jamshed H, Beyl RA, Della Manna DL, et al. Early time-restricted feeding improves 24-hour glucose levels and affects markers of the circadian clock, aging, and autophagy in humans. Nutrients. 2019;11:1234.

Chapter 5
What is the immune system?

The immune system is conceptualized by most people in a similar way as a country's military for defense. If a war breaks out, we can easily visualize a country's military lining up at the border to repel an invading army. Similarly, the immune system is conceptualized to prevent unwanted bacteria or viruses, which are referred to as pathogens, from invading and getting a foothold in the body to cause disease. This is why people conceptualize the need for a strong immune system. While this perspective is not wrong, it is also not correct because immune function is extremely complex and cannot be reduced to having either a weak or strong immune system. It is much more accurate to simplify the complexity of immune function in the context of inflammation.

An anti-inflammatory immune system will eliminate pathogens without an excessive release of symptom-producing inflammatory chemicals, which means that some people can eliminate pathogens without any or just minimal symptoms. This is why healthy people can be exposed to SARS-CoV-2 and be minimally impacted.

In contrast, a pro-inflammatory immune system is less effective at eliminating pathogens and releases an excess of inflammatory chemicals that can produce a host of symptoms, including malaise (feeling unwell), chills, muscle aches, headache, sore throat, cough, fever, difficulty breathing or shortness of breath. Some or all of these symptoms are found in people with the common cold, the seasonal flu, and SARS-CoV-2.

With the above in mind, it should be obvious that we all need an anti-inflammatory immune system. In this book, you will find out how our diets help to determine if we are going to have an anti-inflammatory or pro-inflammatory immune system. Before going into those details, the remainder of this chapter is going to discuss the various cells that make up the immune system.

If you look at your most recent blood test you will see a section entitled CBC (*Complete Blood Count), Platelet Count, and Differential,* or something similar. The Differential section of the lab report lists various immune cells and if they are within or outside the normal range. These immune cells are also called white blood cells and include neutrophils, lymphocytes, monocytes, eosinophils, and basophils. Basic information about these cells can be found at MedlinePlus (1):

Neutrophils

Neutrophils are the most abundant of our immune cells and they primarily protect us against bacteria. When a blood test shows elevated neutrophils, the primary consideration is bacterial infection.

Lymphocytes

Lymphocytes primarily protect us against viruses. When a blood test shows elevated lymphocytes, the primary consideration is a viral infection. There are many different types of lymphocytes, which will be discussed in more detail in Chapters 9 and 11.

Monocytes

Monocytes travel in the blood and are recruited to enter areas of injury and infection. When monocytes arrive, they transform into macrophages, which remove dead cells, damaged tissues, bacteria, and virally-infected cells. Macrophages will be discussed in more detail in Chapter 9.

Eosinophils

Eosinophils defend the body primarily against parasites and bacteria.

Basophils

Basophils release histamine and are the cells involved in allergic reactions and asthma attacks. During allergy season, pollen stimulates basophils to release histamine, which gives people the symptoms of an allergy.

In the absence of an immunosuppressive condition such as AIDS, almost everyone has normal levels of immune cells, which increase according to the nature of the threat, be it bacteria, viral, parasite, or allergens. Whenever immune cells are activated/stimulated to engage an invader, they produce a host of inflammatory chemicals. When produced in excess, these inflammatory chemicals create various symptoms such as aches, pains, fatigue, and the general feeling of unwellness.

The novel coronavirus provides us with the most relevant example of this. People who are exposed to SARS-CoV-2 may have no symptoms, mild symptoms, severe flu-like symptoms, or they may have such severe respiratory symptoms that they die. Same virus but very different symptoms, all of which correlate to the degree to which inflammatory mediators are being released by immune cells in response to the virus.

This means that our attention should NOT be focused on the virus, which we really cannot control; instead, our focus should be on the human body and what causes it to react minimally or severely to a virus. As it turns out, the prevailing inflammatory state of the infected body is the determining factor. A DeFlamed body will have a mild reaction, while an inflamed body will have a more severe reaction, which increases in severity based on the increasing level of inflammation.

References

1. Medline Plus by US government's NIH. https://medlineplus.gov/lab-tests/blood-differential/

Chapter 6
A pro-inflammatory vs a DeFlamed immune system

During the COVID-19 era, it has become more popular than ever for people to speak about strengthening and boosting their immune systems. I have never used that language because it does not reflect how we should view immune function, which I will outline in this chapter.

The immune cells discussed in Chapter 2 have the ability to release pro-inflammatory chemicals and anti-inflammatory chemicals. It should be our goal for our immune systems to be healthy and DeFlamed, which means that immune cells can properly release pro- and anti-inflammatory chemicals based on the needs of the body. When people flame up with a pro-inflammatory diet, their immune cells begin to preferentially release an excess of pro-inflammatory chemicals and simultaneously lose the ability to release anti-inflammatory chemicals. Figure 1 illustrates an anti-inflammatory immune state.

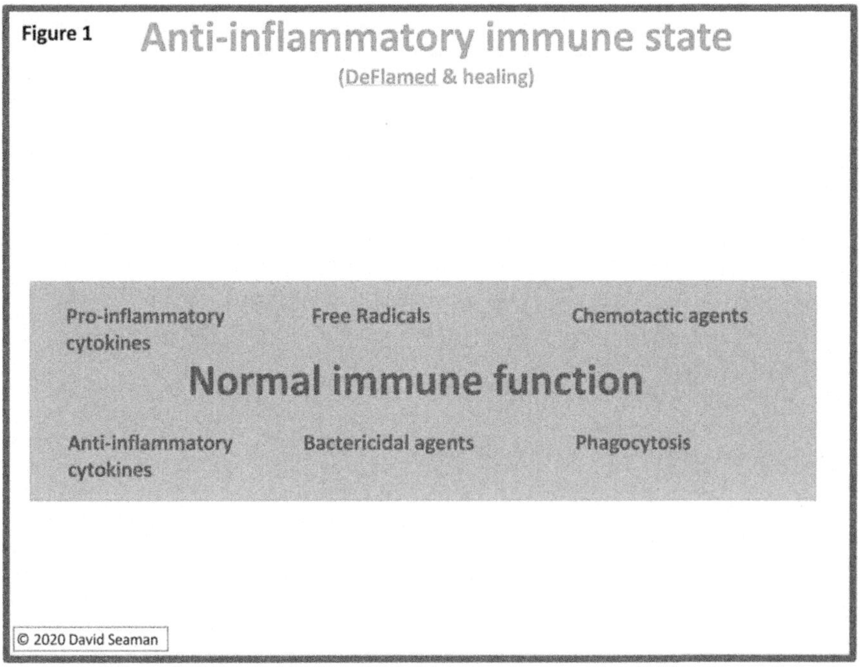

It is not important to understand all the chemicals in Figure 1 at this point. The various chemicals released by immune cells will be discussed in the next chapter. For now, it is important to get the general concept for visualization purposes.

Notice that normal immune function reflects the ability of immune cells to produce pro-inflammatory chemicals (pro-inflammatory cytokines, free radicals, and chemotactic agents) and anti-inflammatory chemicals (anti-inflammatory cytokines and bacteriocidal agents), and also effectively remove damaged cells, bacteria, and viruses by a process called phagocytosis. As stated earlier in this chapter, a normal DeFlamed immune system is responsive to the stressors that impact the body and able to turn on and off inflammation as needed.

In general, healthy, fit, and lean individuals have a DeFlamed immune state, while obese individuals have pro-inflammatory immune state. This is why obese people are at greater risk for developing severe complications when infected by the coronavirus or seasonal flu virus.

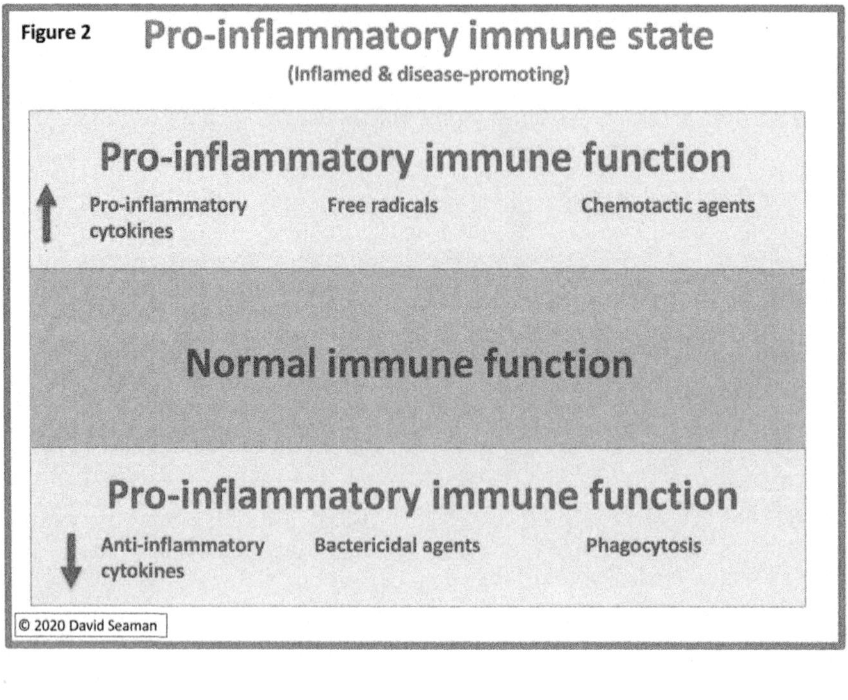

As you can see in Figure 2, a pro-inflammatory immune system produces an excess of pro-inflammatory chemicals and too little anti-inflammatory chemicals. There is an associated reduction in phagocytic capacity, which in the case of a viral infection, this means that the body is less effective at clearing the virus. Figure 2 illustrates this pro-inflammatory shift in immune function.

Figure 2 should help to visualize why it makes no sense to claim that we need to strengthen or boost the immune system. Instead, the conceptual goal should be to DeFlame the immune system so that we reduce the excess production of pro-inflammatory chemicals and increase the production of anti-inflammatory chemicals, and also restore phagocytic and bactericidal activity to normal so pathogens like coronavirus can be eliminated and only deal with mild symptoms during the process. Achieving a normal body weight by eating whole foods is one of the most important things we can do to restore immune function to normal. Obesity and other immune modulating factors will be discussed in upcoming chapters.

Chapter 7
Immune system inflammation chemistry

The material in this chapter about immune chemistry is about the level of an introductory science course in college. In other words, anyone who graduated from high school should be able to understand the information in this chapter, with the understanding that this is not casual reading material. One must focus and concentrate on the material and perhaps review it a couple of times, which is the way we all learned new information in high school, college, and beyond.

Table 1 lists the immune chemistry that was introduced in the last chapter. This by no means represents the totality of immune chemistry, but it will help to properly contextualize immune function in a meaningful fashion so you can understand why a DeFlamed immune system should be the goal. Each of the topics in Table 1 will be discussed in the remainder of this chapter.

Table 1

Pro-inflammatory immune activity	**Anti-inflammatory immune activity**
Pro-inflammatory cytokines	Anti-inflammatory cytokines
Free radicals	Bactericidal agents
Chemotactic agents	Phagocytosis

Before discussing each of the topics in Table 1, it should be understood that we need both pro- and anti-inflammatory immune activity in order to properly deal with injuries and infections. Too little or too much pro- or anti-inflammatory immune activity is problematic. It is important to understand that immune activity needs to be commensurate to our body's needs.

Pro-inflammatory immune activity

In this section, the focus will be about pro-inflammatory cytokines, free radicals and chemotactic agents. Each will be discussed in a context that you should be able to understand to at least appreciate the nature of pro-inflammatory immune function.

What are pro-inflammatory cytokines?

Cytokines are proteins that participate in the inflammatory process. Over 30 cytokines have been identified, most of which are pro-inflammatory. Save for a few, most cytokines are named based on their number. For example, the term interleukin refers to cytokines, which are numbered as interleukin-1, interleukin-2, and so on. The most well-known pro-inflammatory cytokines are interleukin-1 (IL-1), interleukin-6 (IL-6), interleukin-17 (IL-17), and tumor necrosis factor (TNF). These are the cytokines involved in the cytokine storm, which has been discussed in the news and written about in general public magazines in the context of the coronavirus.

If you do an internet search for coronavirus and cytokine storm, you will see multiple articles. The cytokine storm is when cytokine production becomes especially excessive, which can cause certain people to die when they are infected by the coronavirus, flu virus, and other viruses (1,2).

Cytokines are rarely tested for in the clinical setting; however, this is easily remedied by doing a blood test for high sensitivity C-reactive protein (hsCRP). The liver overproduces hsCRP when interleukin-6 (IL-6) is overproduced by immune cells. As outlined in Table 3 in Chapter 4, an hsCRP level below 1 mg/L is normal, between 1-3 mg/L reflects mild to moderate inflammation, and above 3 mg/L reflects high inflammation.

The average middle-aged American has an hsCRP level of 1.5 mg/L and approximately 25% of the population has hsCRP levels greater than 3 mg/L (3). Clearly the average adult American perpetually lives in a state of chronic inflammation to varying degrees, so it should be no wonder why certain people have terrible outcomes when dealing with a viral infection that serves to further increase pro-inflammatory cytokine production.

What should we do? It is important to address all of the known lifestyle factors that increase pro-inflammatory cytokine and hsCRP levels. Consider the fact that a single meal that consists of refined sugar, flour, and fats/oils, causes body cells to produce an excess of pro-inflammatory cytokines and increases hsCRP levels (4). This returns to normal in healthy people after the calories work their way through the bodies. Unfortunately, most people do this several times per day. Indeed, the average American gets almost 60% of their daily calories from these sources, which eventually leads to obesity and chronic high fasting blood glucose levels, both of which are associated with an elevated hsCRP.

The average American has additional lifestyle issues that increase cytokine and hsCRP levels, those being sedentary living, a lack of sleep, mental/emotional stressors, and smoking (3,5). You can see why I think it is foolish to assume that somehow, Bill Gates' coronavirus vaccine is the key intervention we need to return America back to normal.

What are free radicals?

Free radicals are essentially pro-inflammatory oxidizing agents. Consider how old cars are commonly rusted and aged looking. The rusting process is an oxidation process. In the human body, too many free radicals lead to body oxidation, inflammation, physical degeneration, and aging. Our cells produce an excess of free radicals when they are exposed to a pro-inflammatory diet rich in refined sugar, flour, and oils. Our cells also produce an excess of free radicals when we become obese, diabetic, hypertense, and manifest other chronic diseases, such as heart disease, liver disease, cancer, Alzheimer's disease, and Parkinson's disease.

The human body also produces an excess of free radicals when fighting an infection. This is perfectly normal and should be short-lived, with such production returning back to normal after the infection is conquered. The problem is that unhealthy people chronically produce an excess of free radicals. Chapter 11 will explain free radicals in more detail.

<u>What are chemotactic agents?</u>

The word chemotaxis refers to the migration of immune cells to areas of injury or infection. When cells in our bodies are damaged by injury or infection, they release chemotactic agents called chemokines which lead to the recruitment of immune cells into the damaged area for healing purposes. This is a topic that is taught in general physiology classes in college, so it is a widely understood process, but only in the context of injury or infection. It turns out that a pro-inflammatory diet also stimulates chemotaxis, which is best understood by the example of cells in the pancreas that release insulin.

Whenever blood glucose rises, beta cells in the pancreas sense this and release insulin, which allows for the uptake of glucose by muscle cells predominately, and also by fat cells and liver cells. In recent years, it was discovered that these same beta cells also release cytokines and chemokines when they are exposed to high glucose levels.

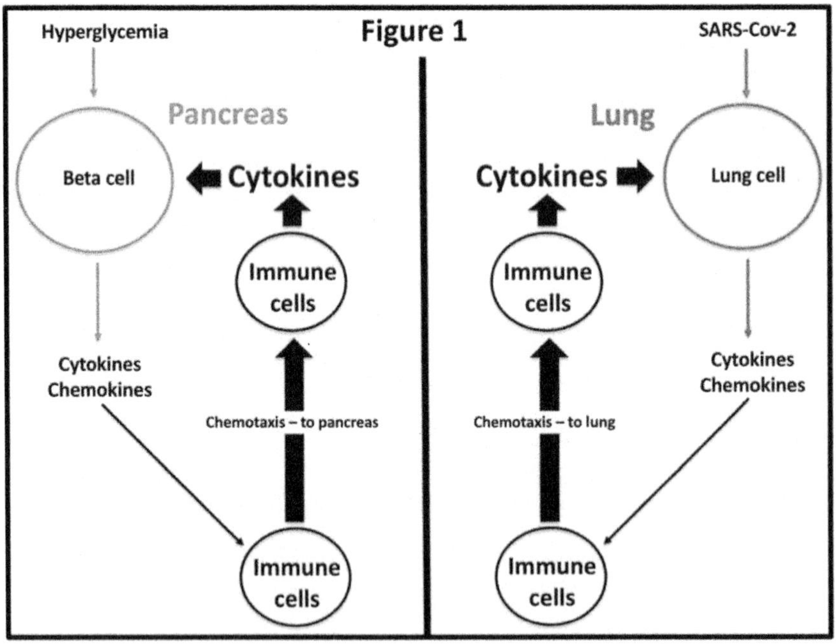

When pancreatic beta cells are exposed to high blood glucose levels (hyperglycemia), they still release insulin AND they also release pro-inflammatory cytokines and chemokines, which is exactly what immune cells do when we suffer from a viral infection. These processes are illustrated in Figure 1, wherein beta cells of the pancreas are stimulated by hyperglycemia, and lung cells, called pneumocytes, are stimulated by the coronavirus known as SARS-CoV-2. Notice in Figure 1 that both beta cells and lung cells release cytokines and chemokines, which causes immune cells to migrate into the pancreas and lungs, respectively, where these newly arriving immune cells begin to release an excess of tissue damaging cytokines (6,7).

Figure 2 was created to illustrate that all body cells flame up when they are exposed to high blood glucose levels. Recall from Chapter 4 that almost 25% of adults between the ages of 40-49 have hyperglycemia (metabolic syndrome) and this rises to over 40% of adults age 60 and older, which means that multiple millions of Americans were already quite flamed up before SARS-CoV-2 arrived on the scene to deliver the final blow to some unfortunate people.

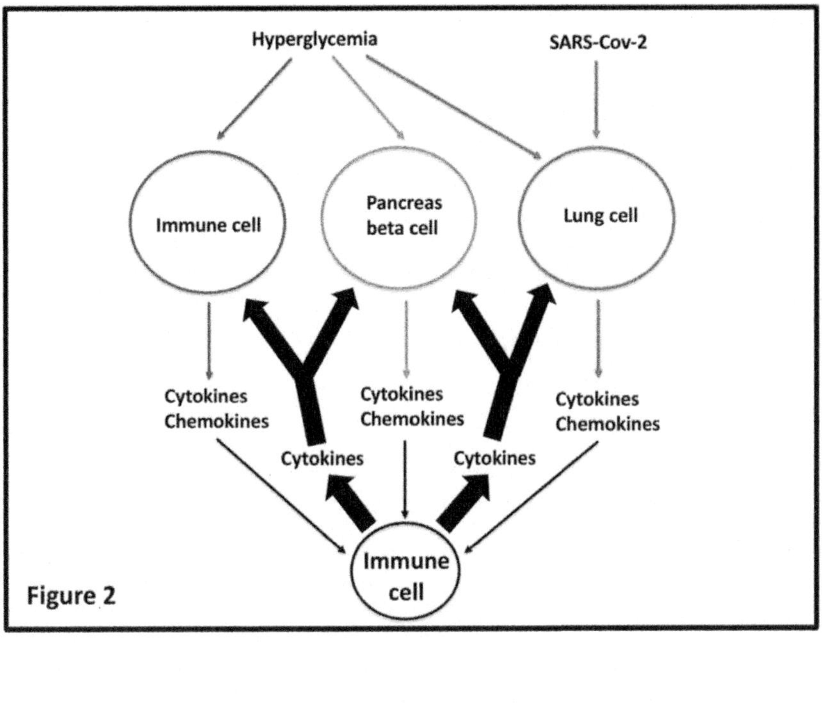

Figure 2

This is why I say that overeating dietary crack (desserts, chips, bread, etc.) causes the human body to become "infected" with sugar. A similar "infection" state occurs during the obesity process, which will be discussed in Chapter 9. It is important to understand that when I use the word "infection" in the context of hyperglycemia and obesity, I am referring to the immune system's response. In both cases, hyperglycemia and obesity create an immune cell profile that resembles a viral infection, which is why obese diabetics are much more likely to have a catastrophic outcome from a coronavirus infection compared to healthy, lean people.

Anti-inflammatory immune chemicals

In this section, the focus will be about anti-inflammatory cytokines, bactericidal agents, and phagocytosis. As with the pro-inflammatory immune chemicals, each will be discussed in a context that you should be able to understand to at least appreciate the nature of anti-inflammatory immune function.

<u>What are anti-inflammatory cytokines?</u>

The key anti-inflammatory cytokine is interleukin-10 (IL-10), which has been referred to as "the master regulator of immunity to infection" (8). Additional anti-inflammatory cytokines include interleukin-4 (IL-4), interleukin-11 (IL-11), and transforming growth factor-ß (TGF-ß).

Our focus will be on IL-10, which is so exceptionally anti-inflammatory that if it gets "boosted" too high, IL-10 will inhibit immune cells from effectively eliminating infective agents from the body (8). This can be likened to watering the plants in a garden; they need water to thrive, but too much water can be damaging. Elevated IL-10 levels should not be a concern for us, as this appears to be more of an issue in the laboratory research setting, wherein scientists can create IL-10 levels higher compared to the patient-care clinical setting wherein reduced IL-10 levels are common.

This is because most patients are overweight or obese and many have the metabolic syndrome or type 2 diabetes, which renders the body less able to produce adequate levels of IL-10 (9-11). In other words, the immune systems of lean, healthy people are better able to produce IL-10 when needed to properly modulate inflammation. It is important to understand that without adequate IL-10, the immune system lives in a perpetual pro-inflammatory state.

Additional diet-related factors are associated with a lower production of IL-10, those being a lack of omega-3 fatty acids, a lack of probiotic bacteria, and a lack of polyphenols from vegetation (12-17). The most robust marker for a reduced capacity to produce IL-10 is a low vitamin D level (18-21).

What are bactericidal agents?

Not well known is that our immune cells produce bacteria-killing (bactericidal) agents. Indeed, our immune cells produce anti-microbial peptides called cathelicidins and defensins, which can lower viral replication rate (21). We also know that cathelicidins exhibit direct antimicrobial activities against a spectrum of microbes, including bacteria, fungi, and viruses (21). It turns out that vitamin D is the key nutrient required for the production of cathelicidins and defensins (21), which means that everyone should identify their vitamin D level and then sunbathe and/or supplement accordingly.

What is phagocytosis?

Macrophages and neutrophils are the two key immune cells that eliminate bacteria and viruses, as well as dead human cells and tissues, from the body. This is achieved via a process called phagocytosis, which is an ancient Greek word that literally means "to eat." These immune cells, called phagocytes, have receptors on their cell membranes that recognize pathogens. This allows phagocytes to engulf (eat) and remove pathogens from the body.

In the case of viruses, an infected cell will express a signaling molecule on its surface, referred to as an "eat-me" signal, which alerts phagocytes to eliminate the infected cell (22). We obviously do not want the capacity of immune cell phagocytosis to be impaired.

Unfortunately, phagocytic activity is impaired in obese individuals (23) and those with type 2 diabetes (24).

Additionally, both obesity and diabetes are inflammatory pathological states associated with hyperglycemia and increased free radical production. Imagine an excess of glucose entering a macrophage, which causes this phagocyte to produce an excess of free radicals. This leads to a depressed ability of the phagocyte to engage in phagocytic activity (25).

To improve immune cell phagocytosis and viral removal, we should all endeavor to normalize the markers of inflammation discussed in Chapter 4. The most notable in the context of phagocytosis includes a normal body mass index (BMI) and waist/hip ratio for tracking obesity, and fasting glucose, postprandial glucose, and hemoglobin A1c for tracking hyperglycemia.

Supplements that have antioxidant functions also offer benefits. This is because, as stated above, an excess production of free radicals by phagocytes reduces their phagocytic capacity (25). Thus, by reducing an excess of free radical production, antioxidant supplements are able to prevent this loss of phagocytic activity. The most studied in this regard is vitamin C (26). Zinc also appears to have a similar effect (27). Our body's antioxidant system will be discussed more in Chapter 11, which will allow for a more detailed appreciation for the possible supplements that work similarly to vitamin C and zinc.

Summary

My hope is that this chapter helped you appreciate that immune function is complex and so, immune system thinking should not be reduced to simple goals like, we need to "boost our immune systems." With this in mind, also understand that while this chapter accurately characterizes key immune functions, it barely scratches the surface of the true scientific complexity of immune function. However, no matter if we view immune function in the fashion described in this chapter or in an extremely complex scientific fashion, understand that our goal should be to DeFlame our bodies so that our immune systems can properly deliver pro- and anti-inflammatory functions as needed to protect us against viral infections.

References

1. Liu Q, Zhou Y, Yang Z. The cytokine storm of severe influenza and development of immunomodulatory therapy. Cell Mol Immunol. 2016;13:3-10.
2. Tisoncik JR, Korth MJ, Simmons CP, et al. Into the eye of the cytokine storm. Microbiol Mol Biol Rev. 2012;76:16-32.
3. Ridker PM. C-reactive protein: simple test to help predict risk of heart attack and stroke. Circulation. 2003;1089:e81-e85.
4. O'Keefe JH, Gheewala NM, O'Keefe JO. Dietary strategies for improving post-prandial gluose, lipids, inflammation, and cardiovascular healthy. J Am Coll Cardiol. 2008;51:249-55.
5. Seaman DR. Body mass index and musculoskeletal pain: is there a connection? Chiro Man Ther. 2013;21:15.
6. Donath MY, Shoelson SE. Type 2 diabetes as an inflammatory disease. Nat Rev Immunol. 2011;11:98-117.
7. Melchjorsen J, Sorensen LN, Paludan SR. Expression and function of chemokines during viral infections: from molecular mechanisms to in vivo function. J Leuk Biol. 2003;74:331-34.
8. Couper KN, Blount DG, Riley EM. IL-10: The master regulator of immunity to infection. J Immunol. 2008;180:5771-77.
9. Van Exel E, Gussekloo J, de Craen AJ, et al. Low production capacity of interleukin-10 associates with the metabolic syndrome and type 2 diabetes. The Leiden 85-plus study. Diabetes. 2002;51:1088-92.
10. Straczkowski M, Kowalska I, Nickolajuk A, et al. Plasman interleukin-10 concentration is positively related to insulin sensitivity in young healthy individuals. Diabetes Care. 2005;28:2036-37.
11. Leon-Cabrera S, Arana-Lechuga Y, Esqueda-Leon E, et al. Reduced systemic levels of IL-10 are associated with severity of obstructive sleep apnea and insulin resistance in morbidly obese humans. Mediators Inflammation. 2015. Article ID: 493409.
12. Ferrucci L, Cherubini A, Bandinelli S et al. Relationship of plasma polyunsaturated fatty acids to circulating inflammatory markers. J Clin Endocrinol Metab. 2006;91(2):439-46.
13. Draper E, Reynolds CM, Canavan M, Mills KH, Loscher CE, Roche HM. Omega-3 fatty acids attenuate dendritic cell function via NF-κB independent of PPARγ. J Nutr Biochem. 2011;22(8):784-90.
14. Sherman PM, Ossa JC, Johnson-Henry K. Unraveling mechanisms of action of probiotics. Nutr Clin Pract. 2009;24:10-14.
15. Erdman SE, Poutahidis T. Probiotic 'glow of health': it's more than skin deep. Benef Microbes. 2014;5:109-19.

16. Yun JM, Jialal I, Devaraj S. Effects of epigallocatechin gallate on regulatory T cell number and function in obese v. lean volunteers. Br J Nutr. 2010;103(12):1771-7.
17. Wong CP, Nguyen LP, Noh SK, Bray TM, Bruno RS, Ho E. Induction of regulatory T cells by green tea polyphenol EGCG. Immunol Lett. 2011;39:7–13.
18. Arnson Y, Amital H, Shoenfeld Y. Vitamin D and autoimmunity: a new aetiological and therapeutic considerations. Ann Rheum Dis. 2007;66:1137-42.
19. Cantorna MT, Mahon BD. Mounting evidence for vitamin D as an environmental factor affecting autoimmune disease prevalence. Exp Biol Med. 2004; 229:1136-42.
20. Cantorna MT, Snyder L, Lin YD, Yang L. Vitamin D and 1,25(OH)2D regulation of T cells. Nutrients. 2015;7:3011-21.
21. Grant WB, Lahore H, McDonnell SL, et al. Evidence that vitamin D supplementation could reduce risk of influenza and COVID-19 infections and deaths. Nutrients. 2020;12:988.
22. Nainu F, Shiratsuchi A, Nakanishi Y. Induction of apoptosis and subsequent phagocytosis of virus-infected cells as an antiviral mechanism. Front Immunol. 2017;8: Article 1220.
23. Morais TC, Honorio-Franca AC, Fujimori M, et al. Melatonin action on the activity of phagocytes from the colostrum of obese women. Medicina. 2019;55:625.
24. Lecube A, Pachon G, Petriz J, Hernandez C, Simo R. Phagocytic activity is impaired in type 2 diabetes mellitus and increases after metabolic improvement. PLoS ONE. 2011;6(8):e23366.
25. Patel V, Dial K, Wu J, et al. Dietary antioxidants significantly attenuate hyperoxia-induced acute inflammatory lung injury by enhancing macrophage function via reducing the accumulation of airway HMGB1. Int J Molec Sci. 2020;21:977.
26. Carr AC, Maggini S. Vitamin C and immune function. Nutrients. 217;9:1211.
27. Gao H, Dai W, Zhao L, Min J, Wang F. The role of zinc and zinc homeostasis in macrophage function. J Immunol Res. 2018; Article ID: 6872621.

Chapter 8
The immune system's acute phase response

It is important to be able to consider pro-inflammatory immune function without focusing on infectious agents like SARS-CoV-2 that causes COVID-19, or the viruses that cause the common cold or seasonal flu. I mentioned this in previous chapters; however, this chapter is devoted completely to this topic. The reason for looking at immune function in this fashion is because it is important to understand that your immune system can make you feel unwell even when you are not infected with a virus or bacteria.

Malaise is a general feeling of unwellness that people equate with coming down with "something," which most commonly turns out to be symptoms that we equate with the common cold. Depending upon how heavy the pollen is in early spring, I may feel malaise, and at that point I cannot tell if it is allergies or a cold. In this case, the symptoms are essentially the same. However, the causes are different; those being pollen or a virus.

This initial state of malaise, and subsequent symptoms, are caused by what is referred to as the acute phase response/reaction. It is the process by which immune cells respond to a stressor and release inflammatory mediators, the most notable being pro-inflammatory cytokines, which causes the liver to produce and release acute phase reactants. C-reactive protein, which was discussed in the previous chapter, is an example of an acute phase reactant. Additional acute phase reactants include angiotensinogen (discussed in Chapter 2), fibrinogen (discussed in the DeFlame breast health book), and many more, including ferritin, serum amyloid A, haptoglobin, alpha1-acid glycoprotein, lipopolysaccharide-binding protein (LBP), alpha1-antitrypsin, hepcidin, vitronectin, and procalcitonin.

The point to understand is that the acute phase response can occur without being infected by a virus. Pollen can cause it, as well as other stressors, such as sleep loss, which will be discussed shortly. This means that when you start to feel unwell, you need to examine your recent activities and identify your stressors so you understand the choices you made that led to the acute phase response so that you make better lifestyle choices in the future.

You should also understand that one can be "infected" with SARS-CoV-2 that causes COVID-19 and have absolutely no acute phase symptoms at all. These are the people who are asymptomatic even though they test positive for SARS-CoV-2. In my view, based on the available evidence, these asymptomatic people have been inappropriately accused of being the primary drivers of the so-called pandemic. While this will likely remain a contentious issue, it appears that infected people who are asymptomatic are NOT likely to be the main transmitters of the virus (1-3).

Consider that in perhaps the first published report about asymptomatic transfer, the authors failed to interview the alleged asymptomatic patient to absolutely confirm that she was asymptomatic (4). This led Dr. Anthony Fauci to triumphantly claim that this study proved that asymptomatic transfer does occur, and it "lays the question to rest" (3). Unfortunately, Dr. Fauci spoke too soon. When the alleged "asymptomatic" patient was questioned, it was discovered that she did have acute phase symptoms when she infected her coworkers. She felt tired, suffered from muscle pain, and was taking Tylenol (3). In short, to date, the prevailing evidence suggests that the presence of a minimal acute phase response is required for viral transmission from one person to another. This contentious subject will be discussed in more detail in Chapter 14.

If everyone in America was infected by SARS-CoV-2 but no one had an acute phase response, no one would have symptoms and the virus would pass through society and go away unnoticed. This means that being infected is not the issue; it is our body's response to the infection that matters.

The acute-phase response can be low-grade, medium-grade or high-grade. A low-grade response leads to feelings of sickness, but no fever or severe illness. A medium-grade response may include a mild fever and worse sickness feelings compared to a low-grade response. In contrast, a high-grade acute phase response can be likened to the cytokine storm discussed in the previous chapter that causes a high fever and other symptoms. In the case of COVID-19, additional symptoms include a severe cough and shortness-of-breath, which can kill people if the high-grade acute phase response is severe enough.

As mentioned above, when we develop the sickness symptoms generated by an acute phase response, we automatically default to thinking that we have some type of infection. This is also how doctors and nurses are trained to view acute phase symptoms. However, mental/emotional and other stressors can create an acute phase response. The best example I can think of is what often happens to students going through final exam week.

I spent almost 15 years teaching chiropractic students. The first school where I taught was on the quarter system and the second was on the trimester system. This means that students had to suffer through a grueling week of final exams 3 and 4 times per year for several years. The week before final exams, students had to attend classes and also take lab exams where they demonstrated diagnosis and treatment procedures. In other words, the last two weeks of a quarter or trimester are highly stressful; students mentally stress about exams, sleep less because of long hours of studying, and they tend to exercise less and eat less healthy due to time constraints.

For most students, the last two weeks of a term are pro-inflammatory, which causes many students to feel unwell compared to the previous weeks of the quarter or trimester due to a low-grade acute phase response. It is not uncommon for some students to develop symptoms that resemble a cold or flu, which leads some to incorrectly believe that they "caught a cold," especially if the term is ending in December during what is commonly called the "cold and flu season." Some just feel unwell and rundown, while others end up spending a few days in bed. Clearly, final exam acute phase reactions do not involve infections or physical injuries; they suffer from mental stressors, a lack of sleep, a disruption of normal routines, lack of exercise, and a more pro-inflammatory diet, which increases cytokine release by immune cells and leads to feelings of sickness as if they were "coming down" with a cold or flu.

In previous chapters, I illustrated how a pro-inflammatory diet and infectious agents stimulate the immune system to create inflammation. It is more difficult to conceptualize how physiologic stressors (sleep loss, sedentary living, and psychosocial stressors) induce inflammation. Scientist have identified that the human body has a signaling system for such stressors, which shift normal physiology and biochemistry into a pro-inflammatory mode. Signaling molecules called alarmins have been identified, which cause immune cells to release inflammatory chemicals, such as cytokines. Figure 1 illustrates how this works by focusing on sleep loss.

HMGB1, stands for high mobility group box-1, which is one of the human body's alarmin molecules that activate the immune system. The HMGB1 alarmin is released by cells that are stressed by sleep loss, sedentary living, and psychosocial stressors that causes immune cells to release pro-inflammatory cytokines (5-7). When this happens, the liver is stimulated to release C-reactive protein, which, as stated earlier in this chapter, is one of many acute phase reactants produced by the liver.

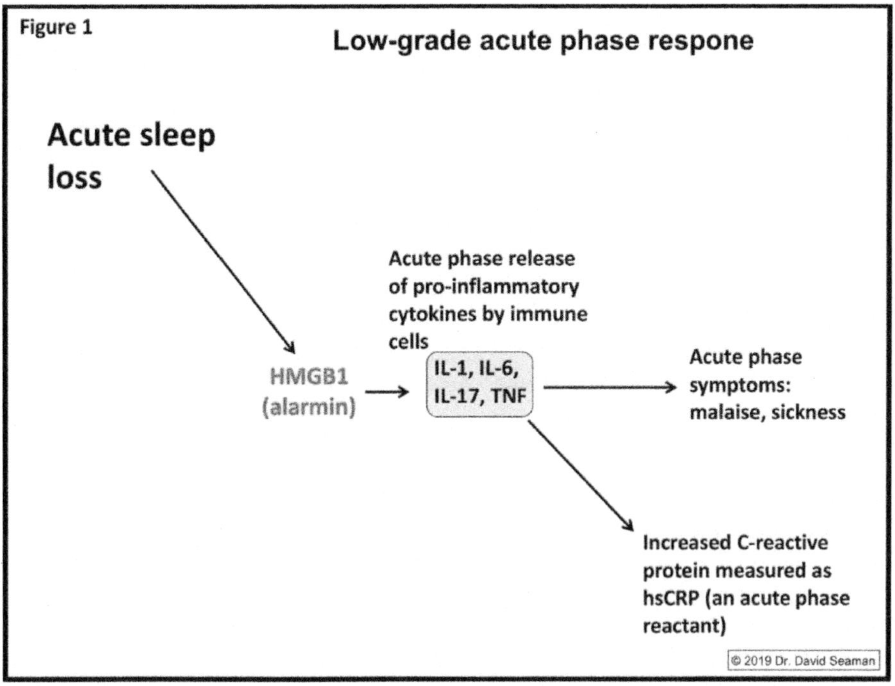

In the clinical setting, HMGB1 and cytokines are not measured to assess a patient's inflammatory status. Instead, high sensitivity C-reactive protein (hsCRP) is used to assess inflammation as discussed in Chapter 7, which is an inexpensive test for inflammation and not surprisingly, it correlates with HMGB1 and pro-inflammatory cytokine levels (8-10).

For a real-life example, imagine how you would feel if you only got 4 hours of sleep per night for the next 10 days. You would likely feel terrible and this is because you would dramatically flame-up, as demonstrated in a 2004 study (11). Subjects were sleep-restricted to 4 hours per night for 10 days and increases in inflammation were tracked by measuring high sensitivity C-reactive protein (hsCRP), which was discussed in the previous chapter. At day one, hsCRP levels were at a normal anti-inflammatory level (less than 1 mg/L); however, by day 10, hsCRP levels rose to 2.75 mg/L (moderate inflammation) to over 4 mg/L (high inflammation) (11).

In summary, just 10 days of sleep loss increases cellular release of HMGB1 that circulates in the blood stream and activates immune cells to release pro-inflammatory cytokines, which stimulate the liver to release an excess of C-reactive protein that corresponds to a level of inflammation that is found in heart disease and depression. This low-grade acute phase response is why we feel unwell if we do not get enough sleep.

While the average person does not suffer from the type of sleep loss used in the study discussed above, we do know that about 1/3 of Americans regularly fail to get adequate sleep. Most of us need 6-9 hours of sleep. This means that if you need 7-8 hours, but only get 6 hours, you will be sleep deprived and suffer from a chronic low-grade acute phase reaction and may feel unwell to some degree on a regular basis.

As stated above, psychosocial stressors and sedentary living also enhance the activation of the HMGB1 alarmin. If you think about the average middle aged or older individual, most don't get enough sleep, most are stressed out by various life issues, and most are sedentary.

In my book, *Weight Loss Secrets You Need To Know*, I outlined how a lack of sleep and psychosocial stressors promote a craving and overconsumption of high calorie comfort foods, most of which are loaded with refined sugar, flour, and oils. This unavoidably leads to the development of obesity and hyperglycemia, both of which also stimulate the HMGB1 alarmin (12,13).

We should understand that the acute phase response symptoms of malaise and feeling sick are a warning signal to our conscious mind that something is wrong with us that needs to be addressed, the most notable being infections and physical injury. Both typically resolve with rest, a comfortable healing environment, adequate fluids, healthy foods, nutritional supplements, and medications. This means that acute phase symptoms should not last very long. However, when we live a pro-inflammatory lifestyle, acute phase symptoms can become chronic, as illustrated in Figure 2.

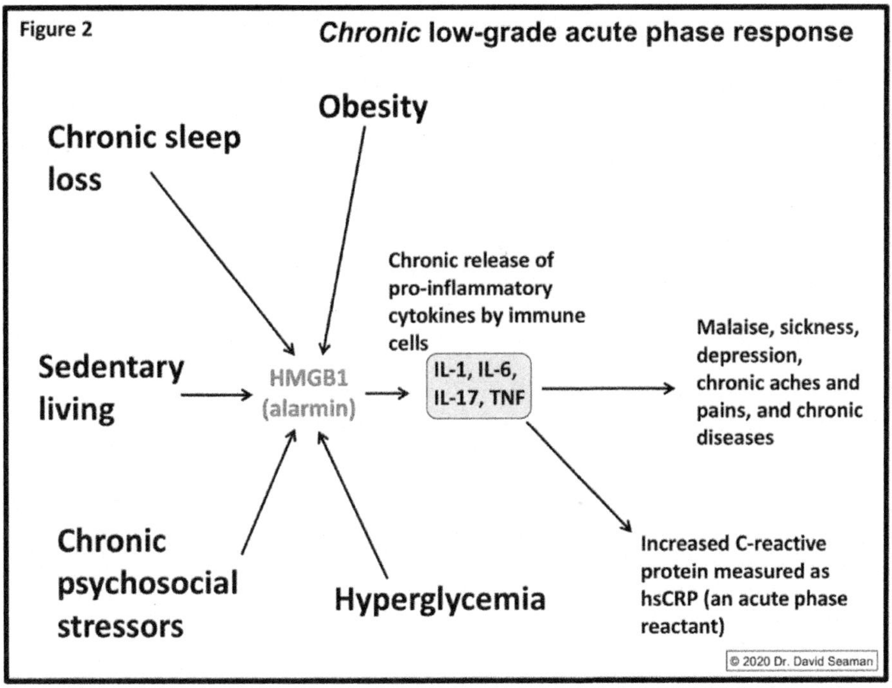

Figure 2 illustrates the activation of the HMGB1 alarmin by sleep loss, psychosocial stressors, sedentary living, obesity, and hyperglycemia. The cumulative effect of these pro-inflammatory lifestyle issues causes people to chronically live in a low-grade acute phase reaction state. These people feel unwell mostly all the time as if they have a low-grade viral infection. They commonly develop chronic muscle/joint pain, and/or headaches, and/or gut pain/distress in their 20s or 30s. By the time they reach 60 years old, many of these people will be diagnosed with a chronic inflammatory disease (heart disease, cancer, Alzheimer's, etc.).

With all the above information in mind, let's again consider the final exam scenario described earlier, with a few modifications. Imagine that you and I, and all of our classmates, were to live alone in environmentally controlled apartments during the final month of a term, such that the air was free of all contaminants and infectious agents, and we had no potential for transferring germs to one another. All of our studying and exam-taking would take place in our single apartments, which means that we have totally controlled the environment for pathogens, pollutants, and allergens. Despite such environmental controls, some students will still suffer from an acute phase response due to the stress of being in a new environment, a lack of normal socializing, adapting to a new lifestyle schedule, less sleep, mentally stressing about finals, less exercising, and whatever else you may think of.

This example should cause you to never forget that malaise and sickness symptoms can have absolutely nothing to do with viruses or bacteria that gain access to our bodies. This example also illustrates that we must identify stressors in our lives and eliminate them to the best of our abilities, because we cannot predict in advance when a new virus will emerge on the scene. And if one does, our goal should be to DeFlame enough so that a new virus, like SARS-CoV-2, will cause at most a mild acute phase response.

References

1. Dr. Maria Van Kerkhove interview. https://www.cnbc.com/2020/06/08/asymptomatic-coronavirus-patients-arent-spreading-new-infections-who-says.html
2. Gao M, Yang L, Chen X, et al. A study on infectivity of asymptomatic SARS-CoV-2 carriers. Respiratory Med. 2020;169:106026. Published on May 13, 2020. https://www.ncbi.nlm.nih.gov/pmc/articles/PMC7219423/
3. Kupferschmidt K. Study claiming new coronavirus can be transmitted by people without symptoms was flawed. Science Magazine. February 3, 2020. https://www.sciencemag.org/news/2020/02/paper-non-symptomatic-patient-transmitting-coronavirus-wrong
4. Rothe C, Schunk M, Sothmann P, et al. Transmission of 2019-nCoV infection from an asymptomatic contact in Germany. N Eng J Med. 2020;382:970-71.
5. Frank MG, Weber MD, Watkins LR, Maier SR. Stress sounds the alarmin: the role of the danger-associated molecular patter HMGB1 in stress-induced neuroinflammatory priming. Brain Behav Immun. 2015;48:1-7.
6. Fleshner M, Frank M, Maier SF. Danger signals and inflammasomes: stress-evoke sterile inflammation in mood disorders. Neuropsychopharmacol. 2017;42:36-45.
7. Goh J, Behringer M. Exercise alarms the immune system: A HMGB1 perspective. Cytokine. 2018;110:222-25.

8. Yao HC, Zhao AP, Han QF, et al. Correlation between serum high-mobility group box-1 and high-sensitivity C-reactive protein and troponin I in patients with coronary artery disease. Exp Ther Med. 2-13;6:121-24.
9. Howren MB, Lamkin DM, Suls J. Associations of depression with C-reactive protein, IL-1, IL-6: a meta-analysis. Psychosomatic Med. 2009;71:171-86.
10. Il'Yasova D, Ivanova A, Morrow JD, et al. Correlation between two markers of inflammation, serum C-reactive protein and interleukin-6, and indices of oxidative stress in patients with high risk of cardiovascular disease. Biomarkers. 2008;13:41-51.
11. Meier-Ewert HK, Ridker PM, Rifai N, et al. Effect of sleep loss on C-reactive protein, an inflammatory marker of cardiovascular risk. J Am Coll Cardiol. 2004;4:678-83.
12. Biscetti F, Rando MM, Nardella E, et al. High mobility group box-1 and diabetes mellitus complications: state of the art and future perspectives. Int J Mol Sci. 2019;20:6258.
13. Zhang J, Zhang L, Zhang S, et al. HMGB1, an innate alarmin, plays a critical role in chronic inflammation of adipose tissue in obesity. Mol Cell Endocrinol. 2017;454:103-111.

Chapter 9
How obesity chemistry resembles viral infection chemistry

As stated earlier in this book, COVID-19 is a health crisis and not a virus crisis. Obesity is perhaps the best example of this fact. As you will read in this chapter, obesity chemistry resembles the immune chemistry of a viral infection.

The obesity pandemic

Approximately 70% of the adult population in the United States is overweight or obese. The CDC (Centers for Disease Control) in Atlanta indicates that the prevalence of obesity was 35.7% among young adults aged 20 to 39 years, 42.8% among middle-aged adults aged 40 to 59 years, and 41.0% among older adults aged 60 and older. In the under 20 age group, almost 20% are obese. Clearly, obesity has reached pandemic proportions in America and a similar trend exists in most other countries. This places most people at a greater risk for developing a chronic disease like heart disease and cancer, and also at a greater risk for developing complications from a viral infection.

Adipose tissue

Adipose tissue is the science term for body fat. Unfortunately, the term body fat creates the misperception that it is only about excess fat created by overeating. It turns out that body fat contains two primary cell types, those being adipocytes (fat cells) and immune cells.

Obese fat cells

Most people do not understand that fat cells are NOT merely cells that store excess calories as fat. In fact, fat cells also produce a variety of substances called adipokines, which include cytokines and other chemicals that are first released within the body fat mass and then gain access to body circulation. Fat cells (adipocytes) can either be lean, overweight, or obese, or in transition among one of these three states, which determines the nature of the chemicals they release.

Lean fat cells produce proper amounts of two key hormones that participate in immune function, those being leptin and adiponectin. As body fat mass increases, fat cells overproduce leptin and underproduce adiponectin, such that obesity is associated with high blood levels of leptin and low adiponectin. Each will be discussed in the following paragraphs.

Leptin

When leptin is overproduced by obese fat cells, it stimulates the immune system to create inflammation (1), which can lead to more severe cases of viral infections. You may recall the swine flu back in 2009, which was called H1N1. To study the effects of obesity on H1N1 infection, scientists overfed mice, which became obese and led to an increased release of leptin. They discovered that high leptin levels were associated with severe cases of H1N1 infection (2). The only way to normalize leptin levels is to lose body fat to the point that all of the inflammation-related markers listed in Chapter 4 become normal.

While it is possible to measure leptin levels, it is not a common test in clinical practice. Fortunately, we know that leptin levels rise in a fashion that is consistent with a rise in body fat mass. Levels of hsCRP (discussed in Chapter 7 and 8) also rise as obesity develops. Additionally, we know that leptin levels rise along with hsCRP (3). In other words, increasing leptin levels generally correlate to increasing hsCRP levels, so we really just need to keep track of our hsCRP levels (3).

Adiponectin

As stated above, in contrast to leptin, which is overproduced by obese fat cells, adiponectin is underproduced. Lean fat cells produce proper amounts of adiponectin, which is then released into body circulation to deliver multiple anti-inflammatory functions. In short, adiponectin DeFlames multiple organs, including skeletal muscle, liver, brain, heart, and pancreas (4). Adiponectin also DeFlames immune cells (4,5), which means that adequate levels of adiponectin DeFlames the immune system.

As body fatness increases, there is a commensurate reduction in adiponectin production, and therefore, less adiponectin in circulation and less anti-inflammatory activity throughout the body. Consequently, pro-inflammatory immune activity is enhanced. In other words, obese individuals have elevated levels of leptin and reduced levels of adiponectin, so it should not be a surprise that obese individuals have an increased susceptibility to viral infections, prolonged viral shedding, and a delay in the resolution of a viral infection (6). For this reason, scientists have concluded that, "quarantine in obese subjects should likely be longer than normal weight individuals." (6)

In summary, obese fat cells are pro-inflammatory compared to lean fat cells, which puts obese people at a greater risk for developing a viral infection and suffering from complications compared to lean individuals. In the next section, you will see how obese body fat immune cells further increase these risks.

Obese body fat immune cells

One of the first studies that identified immune cells in adipose tissue was published in 2003 (7). This is an extremely new finding in science and changes the way we should look at body fatness. The historical view was that overweight or obese individuals were merely viewed as carriers of excess stored calories. Now we know that adipose tissue is an organ, comprised of two major cell types, those being adipocytes (described above) and immune cells, each of which produces numerous chemicals that influence local adipose tissue physiology and systemic (full body) physiology.

The term "adipose tissue remodeling" is used to describe the transformation of lean adipose tissue that contains healthy anti-inflammatory fat and immune cells to obese adipose tissue with pro-inflammatory fat and immune cells (8). It is important to understand that the immune cell profile in obese remodeled adipose tissue resembles that of a viral infection or autoimmune disease. I personally think we should view obesity as a state of being "infected" by excess calories, to which the immune system responds accordingly by releasing a host of pro-inflammatory chemicals, which would otherwise be released only if there is an actual bacterial or viral infection. This is outlined in Figure 1 on the next page.

A point of clarification before continuing…it is a mistake to think that our stored fat comes mostly from the fat we eat. In fact, the majority of calories we eat come from refined sugar and flour, which makes up approximately 40% of all the calories Americans consume. The excess sugar/flour calories we eat are converted into *saturated* fat and stored in adipocytes. This means that obese fat cells are packed with stored saturated fat, which mostly comes from overeating refined sugar and flour. For more information about saturated fat, unsaturated fat, trans fat, and cholesterol, check out *The DeFlame Diet* book that contains 60 pages about these topics.

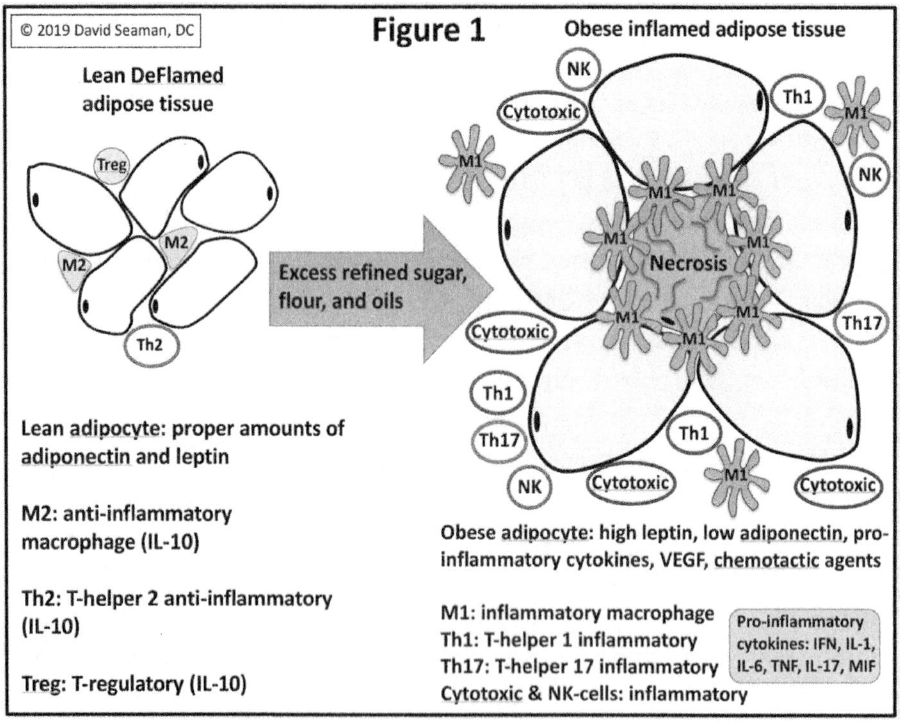

There are two key immune-activating events that occur as adipocytes fill up with fat. One involves a reduction in oxygen levels within the adipose tissue mass, referred to as hypoxia. The hypoxia causes adipocytes to release chemotactic agents (chemokines were discussed in Chapter 7), which attract immune cells to enter the hypoxic fat mass (8,9). The second key event is the release of fat from obese fat cells.

As obese fat cells age, they become necrotic (cell death) and literally go through a rotting process. These rotting fat cells release their great abundance of stored saturated fatty acids. It turns out that the receptor for microbial antigens (infective proteins) on immune cells, called a Toll-like receptor-4 (TLR4), also responds to the saturated fatty acids that are released by rotting fat cells (9). This means that non-microbial factors are capable of activating the immune system to behave like a chronic low-grade viral infection is present – in the case of the majority of Americans, we become chronically "infected," not by viruses or bacteria, but by excess calories from sugar, flour, and refined oils. This is why obese people feel unwell, and this obviously becomes worse if one is actually infected by a virus, such as the common cold, seasonal flu, or SARS-CoV-2 that causes COVID-19.

One of the immune cells found in obese adipose tissue is called a macrophage, the previously discussed phagocyte, whose function is to engulf bacteria and virus-infected cells; however, there are no infectious microbes in body fat. The macrophages show up in abundance to engulf the fat-laden and rotting adipocytes, as if they were bacteria or virus-infected cells.

You can see in Figure 1, which is nicely colorized in the Kindle version of this book, the difference in immune cell types that make up lean adipose tissue and obese adipose tissue (10-13). Notice how fat cells swell in size as they take in calories and become obese. Also notice how the immune cell population completely changes when lean fat cells are transformed into obese fat cells, and M1 macrophages encircle the necrotic fat cell to create what looks like a crown. Scientists have examined the structural relationship between necrotic fat cells and macrophages, which is referred to as a crown-like structure (14).

Notice also in Figure 1 that lean adipose tissue contains three different anti-inflammatory immune cells, all of which release the extremely important anti-inflammatory cytokine called interleukin-10 (IL-10) that was discussed previously in Chapter 7. The anti-inflammatory macrophage is designated as M2. The other two cells are anti-inflammatory T lymphocytes. One is called a T-helper 2 cell (Th2). The second is a T-regulatory cell (Treg), which releases anti-inflammatory IL-10 and also functions to promote self-tolerance, which means they prevent autoimmune disease expression.

Clearly, we all need to have lean anti-inflammatory adipose tissue. Unfortunately, during the obesity process, anti-inflammatory fat cells and immune cells are replaced by those that are pro-inflammatory and capable of perpetually releasing pro-inflammatory chemistry 24 hours per day, which is augmented whenever excess calories are consumed.

The obese adipose tissue illustrated in Figure 1 should scare you…it scares me for sure. Life is difficult enough on so many levels for the average person that no one should self-impose an additional layer of misery on themselves by moving through life with rotting fat cells in their bodies that behave biochemically in a fashion that resembles a viral infection.

Th1 cells (T-helper 1 cells) typically participate in autoimmune disease expression, with rheumatoid arthritis and psoriasis being the most well-known. Th1 cells release a cytokine called interferon (IFN) which causes neighboring immune cells, particularly M1 macrophages, to release their pro-inflammatory cytokines (IL-1, IL-6, TNF). When IFN was used to treat patients with chronic active hepatitis C, 40% of subjects developed full-blown major depression (15).

Th17 (T-helper 17 cells) were discovered more recently compared to Th1 and Th2 cells. They were named based on their release of interleukin-17 (IL-17), another pro-inflammatory cytokine. The main role of IL-17 in humans is to combat bacterial, fungal, and viral infections (16,17); however, Th-17 cells rapidly accumulate in obese adipose tissue (12), which, as stated above, is "infected" with excess calories and not microorganisms.

Cytotoxic T-cells and natural killer (NK) cells typically show up to release pro-inflammatory cytokines to combat cancer and viral infections. This information should again alert you to the fact that the human body perceives obesity as a biochemical state that resembles a chronic viral infection. No one should be surprised why obese individuals with rotting fat cells are far more likely to be fatigued, lethargic, depressed, and in physical pain compared to their lean counterparts, AND far more likely to have a catastrophic outcome if infected by SARS-CoV-2 or any other virus.

The pro-inflammatory transformation illustrated in Figure 1 occurs anywhere that obese fat cells become hypoxic and necrotic. Unfortunately, the average American (70% of us) is either overweight or obese, which means that most Americans are literally rotting to death. Stated in a more scientific way, this means that adipose tissue is remodeled to varying degrees in all of these individuals and resembles, to varying degrees, the pro-inflammatory adipose tissue image in Figure 1. In this state, obese adipose tissue perpetually releases pro-inflammatory cytokines into body circulation by which they promote inflammation as if they were infected by a virus. This means that the average obese person walks around 24 hours per day in a low-grade viral infection state of body chemistry.

Based on the information in this chapter, no one should be surprised or take it as a personal attack when scientists concluded that, "quarantine in obese subjects should likely be longer than normal weight individuals" (6). As stated earlier in this chapter, obese people have an increased susceptibility to viral infections, prolonged viral shedding, and a delay of resolution of a viral infection (6).

Steps to take to get obesity under control

Many people do not realize how overweight or obese they actually are. My suggestion is to do an internet search for "BMI NIH," which will take you the NIH's website where you can insert your height and weight to calculate your body mass index (BMI). Your goal is for your BMI to be below 25. Next, you want to check your waist/hip ratio and make sure, if you are a woman, yours is below .8, and if you are a man, yours is below .95.

You should also read *Weight Loss Secrets You Need To Know*, which outlines how to mentally get control of your eating, commonly called mindfulness. All the key barriers and challenges to effective weight management are presented in a fashion that will allow you to become the master of your eating environment.

It is not just important to control your caloric intake in general and to specifically eliminate calories from refined sugar, flour, and oil. You also need to dramatically increase your consumption of vegetation, which are loaded with vitamins, minerals, and anti-inflammatory pigments called polyphenols/carotenoids (see the chapter on polyphenols/carotenoids in *The DeFlame Diet* book for more information).

Not surprisingly, exercise is very important for weight management; however, there is a better way to view exercise…it is an extremely anti-inflammatory activity so long as you exercise within your individual tolerance zone. Too little exercise is not enough for DeFlaming purposes and too much can be pro-inflammatory.

Consider, for example, that exercise training reduces the expression of TLR4 (the Toll-like receptor described above) on immune cells, which helps to down-regulate the inflammatory state (18). Exercise also reduces oxidative stress (excess free radical production) and improves mitochondrial function so that fats and ketones can be readily used as energy (18).

Exercise also increases the body's production of IL-10, the powerful anti-inflammatory cytokine described earlier, and reduces immune cell production of TNF (18). There is also evidence from an obese animal model that exercise can promote the switch from a pro-inflammatory M1 macrophage population to the anti-inflammatory M2 macrophage in adipose tissue (19). Clearly, we should all be engaged in regular exercise.

Dental health is a final consideration that overweight and obese individuals should take seriously, as this population is far more likely to manifest dental disease (20). Obviously, dental health should be taken seriously by everyone. It is just that periodontal disease is more common in the overweight and obese populations (20). In the context of viral infections, notice the title of a recent article:

> Sampson V, Kamona N, Samspon A. Could there be a link between oral hygiene and the severity of SARS-CoV-2 infections? Brit Dent J. 2020;228:971-75.

In this article, the scientists explain that pro-inflammatory cytokines, such as IL-1 and TNF, from periodontally diseased tissues can enter saliva and be aspirated to cause inflammation or infection of the lungs. Therefore, inadequate oral hygiene can increase the risk of inter-bacterial exchanges between the mouth and lungs, and thus, increase the risk of respiratory infections. In other words, we should all be flossing and brushing daily and see a dentist for regular cleanings.

References

1. Naylor C, Petri WA. Leptin regulation of immune responses. Trends Mol Med. 2-16;22:88-98.
2. Zhang Aj, To KK, Lau CL, et al. Leptin mediates the pathogenesis of severe 2009 pandemic influenza A (H1N1) infection associated with cytokine dysregulation in mice with diet-induced obesity. J Infect Dis. 2013;207:1270-80.

3. Hribal ML, Fiorentino TV, Sesti G. Role of C reactive protein (CRP) in leptin resistance. Curr Pharm Design. 2014;20:609-15.
4. Xu A, Wang Y, Lam KS. Adiponectin. In: Fantuzzi G, Mazzone T, Eds. Adipose tissue and adipokines in health and disease. Totowa, NJ: Human Press; 2007: p.47-59.
5. Luo Y, Liu M. Adiponectin: a versatile player of innate immunity. J Mol Cell Biol. 2016;8:120-28.
6. Luzi L, Radaelli MG. Influenza and obesity: its odd relationship and the lessons for COVID-19 pandemic. Acta Diabetologica. 2020; April 5. Epub ahead of print.
7. Weisberg SP, McCann D, Desai M, et al. Obesity is associated with macrophage accumulation in adipose tissue. J Clin Invest. 2003;112:1796-1808.
8. Sun K, Kusminski CM, Scherer PE. Adipose tissue remodeling and obesity. J Clin Invest. 2011;121:2094-2101.
9. Ferrante AW. The immune cells in adipose tissue. Diabetes Obes Meta. 2013;15:34-38.
10. Harford KA, Reynolds CM, McGillicuddy FC, Roche HM. Fats, inflammation and insulin resistance: insights to the role of macrophage and T-cell accumulation. In adipose tissue. Proc Nutr Soc. 2011;70:408-17.
11. Cautivo KM, Molofsky AB. Regulation of metabolic health and adipose tissue function by group 2 innate lymphoid cells. Eur J Immunol. 2016;46:1315-25.
12. Chehimi M, Vidal H, Eljaafari A. Pathogenic role of IL-17-producing immune cells in obesity, and related inflammatory disease. J Clin Med. 2017;6:68.
13. Reilly SM, Saltiel AR. Adapting to obesity with adipose tissue inflammation. Nat Rev Endocrinol. 2017;13:633-43.
14. Murano I, Barbatelli G, Parisani V, et al. Dead adipocytes, detected as crown-like structures, are prevalent in visceral fat depots of genetically obese mice. J Lipid Res. 2008;49:1562-68.
15. Bonaccorso S, Meltzer H, Maees M. Psychological and behavioral effects of interferons. Curr Opin Psychiatry. 2000;13:673-677.
16. Yang B, Kang H, Fung A, et al. The role of interleukin-17 in tumour proliferation, angiogenesis, and metastasis. Mediators Inflamm. 2014:623759.
17. Crow CR, Chen K, Pociask DA, et al. Critical role of IL-17RA in immunopathology of influenza infection. J Immunol. 2009;183:5301-10.
18. Kruger K. Inflammation during obesity – pathophysiological concepts and effects of physical activity. Dtsch Z Sportmed. 2017;68:163-69.
19. Kawanishi N, Yano H, Yokogawa Y, Suzuki K. Exercise training inhibits inflammation in adipose tissue via both suppression of macrophage infiltration and acceleration of phenotypic switching from M1 to M2 macrophages in high-fat-diet-induced obese mice. Exerc Immunol Rev. 2010;16:105-18.
20. Martinez-Herrera M, Silvestre-Rangil J, Silvestre FJ. Association between obesity and periodontal disease. A systematic review of epidemiological studies and controlled clinical trials. Med Oral Patol Oral Cir Bucal. 2017;22:e708-15.

Chapter 10
How vitamin D deficiency creates viral infection chemistry

As you read in the previous chapter, as our body fat mass becomes obese, fat cells begin to function in a pro-inflammatory fashion and anti-inflammatory immune cells are replaced by pro-inflammatory immune cells. This can lead many to believe that their immune systems are anti-inflammatory if they are not overweight or obese, which is not necessarily true.

It is certainly possible for me to eat 60% of my calories from refined sugar, flour, and omega-6 oils, and still keep my overall caloric intake at a level that does not cause me to gain weight. If I did this, I would still be deficient in key nutrients such as potassium, magnesium, iodine, omega-3 fatty acids, polyphenols, carotenoids, and assuming I avoided sun exposure, I would also be deficient in vitamin D. If I were to do this, then my immune system would behave in a pro-inflammatory fashion that is similar to that which occurs in obese adipose tissue. Vitamin D deficiency provides us with the best example of this shift to a pro-inflammatory state.

Vitamin D deficiency and related supplementation has become extremely popular in the last 15-20 years. Research has identified that multiple diseases are promoted by a chronic deficiency of vitamin D. Table 1 below is from *The DeFlame Diet* book, which highlights many of the conditions related to a deficiency of vitamin D. Notice that the first four conditions in the left column demonstrate the importance of vitamin D for dealing with viruses and bacteria.

Table 1 - Potential consequences of vitamin D deficiency

Influenza	Muscle aches
Common cold	Schizophrenia
Tuberculosis	Depression
Bacterial vaginosis	Metabolic syndrome
Rickets	Type 2 diabetes
Osteomalacia (bone pain)	Osteoarthritis

Back pain	Muscle weakness
Pseudofractures	Osteoporosis
Widespread pain	Ulcerative colitis
Asthma	Rheumatoid arthritis
Cardiovascular disease	Parkinson's disease
Hypertension	Alzheimer's
Epilepsy	Breast cancer
Type 1 diabetes	Prostate cancer
Multiple sclerosis	Colon cancer
Crohn's disease	Pancreatic cancer

Like obesity, a lack of vitamin D increases inflammation by increasing the number of pro-inflammatory immune cells in circulation that release the various pro-inflammatory cytokines that promote the acute phase response. So, if a person is obese and hyperglycemic, and also vitamin D deficient, which is quite common, then the vitamin D deficiency state will augment the pro-inflammatory state of obesity and hyperglycemia. If one is not obese, but is deficient in vitamin D, this will lead to an increased number of pro-inflammatory immune cells and a reduction of anti-inflammatory immune cells in body circulation.

Figure 1 in this chapter illustrates the same pro- and anti-inflammatory T-lymphocytes that were discussed in the previous chapter about obesity. Th0 cells are T-helper precursor cells, which differentiate into T-helper 1 cells (Th1), T-helper 2 cells (Th2), T-helper 17 cells (Th17), and T-regulatory cells (Treg).

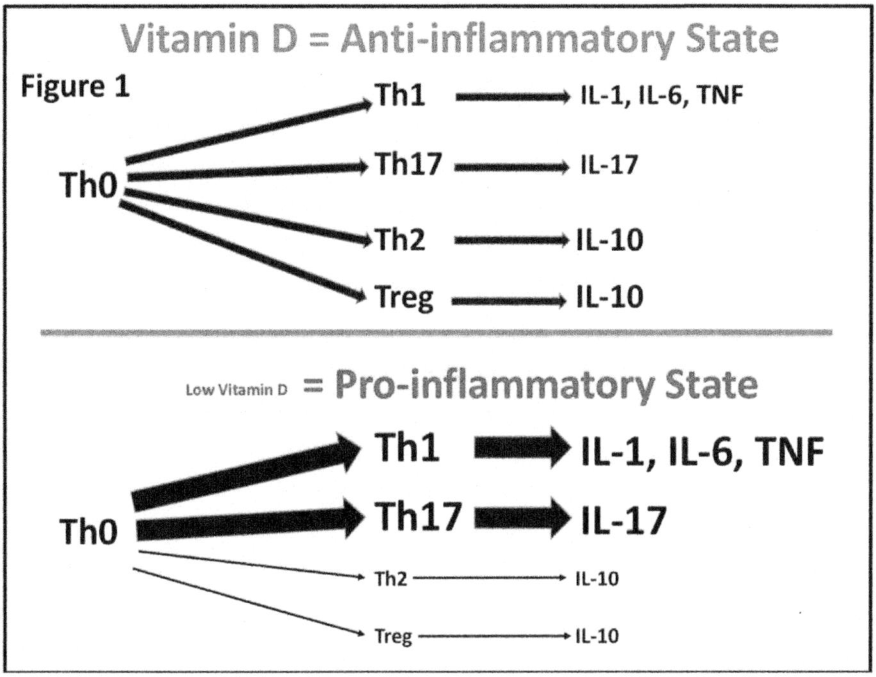

Th1 and Th17 cells promote inflammation by releasing pro-inflammatory cytokines, such as interleukin-1 (IL-1), interleukin-6 (IL-6), interleukin-17 (IL-17), and tumor necrosis factor (TNF). Th2 and Treg cells inhibit inflammation by releasing interleukin-10 (IL-10), the key anti-inflammatory cytokine discussed in previous chapters. For a normal, healthy DeFlamed state of immunity, we need a proper balance between the pro-inflammatory and anti-inflammatory cells and their respective cytokines.

When there is an imbalance in cytokine production, it is never shifted toward being too anti-inflammatory, which means the balance problem always shifts toward being pro-inflammatory. This means that we should not engage in behaviors that inhibit our anti-inflammatory T-cells to shift us into a pro-inflammatory state that can lead to the development of a cytokine storm in some people.

From a practical perspective, we can generally view any unhealthy lifestyle choice as a promoter of pro-inflammatory immune responses and an inhibitor of anti-inflammatory immune responses. Obesity provides us with an example of this pro-inflammatory shift in immune function, as illustrated in the previous chapter. Similarly, vitamin D and immune cell function has been studied by scientists, so we can create a visual image of pro-inflammatory immune cell expression when there is an inadequate level of vitamin D (1-3).

Notice in Figure 1 that Th0 cells are the precursors to all the other T-cells. Th0 cells are referred to as naïve cells, which have the capacity to become both anti-inflammatory Th2 and Treg cells, or pro-inflammatory Th1 and Th17 cells. Notice that when there is adequate vitamin D, we get a balanced production of T-cells. However, when we are deficient in vitamin D, Th0 cells are converted into pro-inflammatory T-cells. This is especially problematic in the context of viral infections, as Th1 and Th17 cells are activated during viral infections (4-6). This means that a vitamin D deficiency state represents a biochemical state of viral infection, which only gets augmented if a virus shows up.

If this was not bad enough, we also know that an inadequate intake of magnesium and omega-3 fatty acids creates a similar pro-inflammatory immune cell profile as obesity and vitamin D deficiency (7,8). In other words, we suffer cumulative pro-inflammatory "hits" when we adopt an unhealthy lifestyle, all of which predisposes one to develop a severe case of COVID-19.

Not only does vitamin D promote an anti-inflammatory balance of T-cells as described above, it is also directly involved in pathogen killing. Recall from Chapter 7 that vitamin D is required by immune cells to produce anti-microbial peptides called cathelicidins and defensins, which can lower viral replication rates (9). We also know that cathelicidins exhibit direct antimicrobial activities against a spectrum of microbes, including bacteria, fungi, and viruses (9). Clearly, everyone should identify their vitamin D level and then sunbathe and/or supplement accordingly.

Most experts agree that we should get our vitamin D level tested, as measured by 25(OH)D in a blood test. The goal, as described in *The DeFlame Diet* book, should be to reach 70 ng/ml.

References

1. Cantorna MT, Mahon BD. Mounting evidence for vitamin D as an environmental factor affecting autoimmune disease prevalence. Exp Biol Med. 2004; 229:1136-42.
2. Cantorna MT, Snyder L, Lin YD, Yang L. Vitamin D and 1,25(OH)2D regulation of T cells. Nutrients. 2015;7:3011-21.
3. Arnson Y, Amital H, Shoenfeld Y. Vitamin D and autoimmunity: a new aetiological and therapeutic considerations. Ann Rheum Dis. 2007;66:1137-42.
4. Yang B, Kang H, Fung A, et al. The role of interleukin-17 in tumour proliferation, angiogenesis, and metastasis. Mediators Inflamm. 2014:623759.
5. Crow CR, Chen K, Pociask DA, et al. Critical role of IL-17RA in immunopathology of influenza infection. J Immunol. 2009;183:5301-10.
6. Maloy KJ, Burkhart C, Junt TM. Cd4+ cell subsets during virus infection: protective capacity depends on effector cytokine secretion and on migratory capability. J Exp Med. 2000;191:2159-70.
7. Chung HS, Park CS, Hong SH, et al. Effects of magnesium pretreatment on the levels of T helper cytokines and on the severity of reperfusion syndrome in patients undergoing living donor liver transplantation. Magnesium Res. 2013;26:46-55.
8. Hichami A, Grissa O, Mrizak I, et al. Role of T-cell polarization and inflammation and their modulation by n-3 fatty acids in gestational diabetes and macrosomia. J Nutr Metab. 2016; Article ID:3124960.
9. Grant WB, Lahore H, McDonnell SL, et al. Evidence that vitamin D supplementation could reduce risk of influenza and COVID-19 infections and deaths. Nutrients. 2020;12:988.

Chapter 11
Free radicals and the antioxidant system in the context of viral infections

Supplementation with vitamins C and D, as well as zinc, became especially popular during the COVID-19 crisis. It was discussed on television news shows, in YouTube videos, and in print/internet media. The general perception I came away with in many cases is that people perceive these nutrients to be key for immune function, which is not correct. These and other nutrients are important for cells in general and not because they have special anti-viral or immune-boosting properties.

Zinc provides us with an excellent example to illustrate how health benefits of so-called "immune boosting" nutrients has been misrepresented. Scientists have clearly demonstrated that the concentration of zinc required to kill viruses far exceeds the level we can achieve from a healthy diet and zinc supplementation (1). So why would we be told to supplement with zinc and vitamins C and D to help fight COVID-19? The same reason why people with vision loss due to macular degeneration are told to take the exact same supplements (2,3); to reduce oxidative stress (free radicals) and inflammation. To demonstrate that this is true, consider this study about zinc supplementation in men and women aged 55-87 years that was inclusive for all ethnic groups (4).

A total of fifty subjects took either 45 mg of zinc per day or a placebo for one year. The study was double-blind and placebo-controlled, which means that the subjects and scientists did not know which 25 subjects received zinc and which 25 subjects received the placebo. At the end of the year study period, it was determined that only 29% of subjects taking zinc had infections, while 88% of those taking the placebo had infections. The reason for this is because those taking the zinc had significantly reduced oxidative stress and pro-inflammatory cytokines (4), which made them significantly less likely to have an acute phase response to viruses and other stressors during that one-year period.

With the above in mind, we should understand the biochemical benefits of zinc without focusing on viral infections, macular degeneration, or other conditions. Zinc is part of an important antioxidant enzyme called superoxide dismutase, which reduces a free radical called superoxide that is designated as O_2- (5). As illustrated in Figure 1, zinc (Zn) also inhibits a pro-inflammatory signaling molecule called nuclear factor kappa-B (NF-kB), which leads to less pro-inflammatory cytokine production (6).

The information in the previous paragraph is likely to contain words that are not familiar to you. Learning new things can be particularly annoying for adults. I recently transformed my yard into a miniature food forest, which took me about two years to complete. I planted dozens of trees, during which time I learned how to improperly and then properly plant and water-in a new tree. I also had to learn the many facets of tree care, insect control, weed control, pruning, and fertilizer use. Many of the words I learned during this process were new to me, but I had to go through the process to become somewhat proficient at managing my transformed yard.

I also had to work through the annoyance and frustration of dealing with different, and sometimes contradictory, recommendations I received at various nurseries and in the garden section of stores like Lowes and Home Depot. I mostly felt dumb through the process but stuck with it. Now I am less ignorant and less frustrated and can look at my yard and visualize how to plant it with pollinators and food trees. I tell you this story because this chapter will likely be the most confusing because of the biochemistry, but you need to stick with it to develop an understanding about free radicals and inflammation.

While Figure 1 on the next page likely looks daunting at first glance, it is not difficult to understand so don't panic. You may have to read this chapter a few times, which is normal; and remember, this is how learning works.

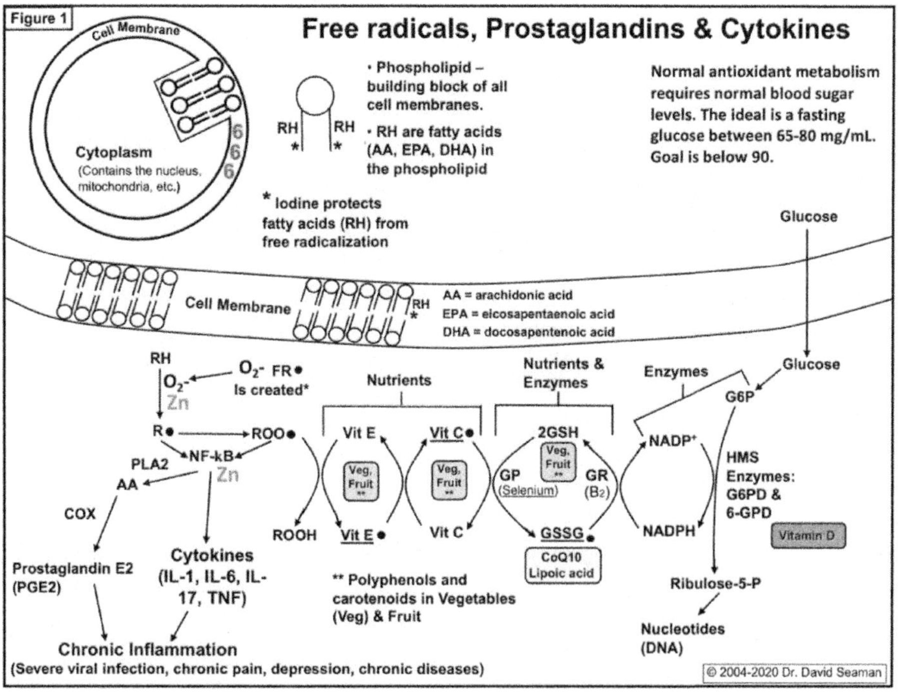

The first thing to do is look at the abbreviations in Figure 1. Then look at Table 1 below and you will see descriptions for each. Spend a little time familiarizing yourself with the abbreviations and the descriptions. Then only look at the abbreviations and test yourself to see if you can remember the descriptions. Make a game out of this if you can. Force your brain to do it even though it may be frustrating.

When you understand this chapter and familiarize yourself with the language and concepts, you will understand how diet causes inflammation at a level higher than most people you know, and you will also understand why people become reliant on medications with unwanted side effects (Table 2).

Table 1 - Key to Figure 1

Abbreviations	Descriptions
Zn	Zinc
O_2-	Superoxide free radical
•	Free radical designation
RH	Fatty acid in phospholipid, also called a lipid

R•	Fatty acid radical or lipid radical
ROO•	Lipid peroxyl radical
Vit E•	Vitamin E radical
Vit C•	Vitamin C radical
2GSH	Reduced glutathione (an antioxidant made by the body)
GSSG•	Oxidized or "free radicalized" glutathione
GP	Glutathione peroxidase (antioxidant enzyme that requires selenium)
GR	Glutathione reductase (antioxidant enzyme that requires riboflavin [vitamin B2])
NF-kB	Nuclear Factor-kappa B (key inflammation signaling molecule)
PLA2	Phospholipase A2 (enzyme that clips fatty acids off of phospholipids to promote or reduce inflammation). PLA2 is inhibited by corticosteroids.
COX	Cyclooxygenase (enzyme that converts arachidonic acid [AA] in prostaglandin E2 [PGE2]. COX is inhibited by anti-inflammatory drugs (aspirin, ibuprofen, Tylenol, etc.)
AA	Arachidonic acid (an omega-6 fatty acid found in excess in meat, fish, chicken that was fed a grain-based diet)
EPA	Eicosapentaenoic acid (an omega-3 fatty acid found in fish oil, cold water fish, and any animal that eats green vegetation – such as grass-fed cattle)
DHA	Docosahexaenoic acid (an omega-3 fatty acid found in fish oil, cold water fish, and any animal that eats green vegetation – such as grass-fed cattle)

Notice in Table 1 that PLA2 and COX are enzymes that lead to the production of prostaglandin E2 (PGE2). PLA2 clips diet-derived arachidonic acid from a cell membrane phospholipid. When this happens the COX enzyme converts diet-derived arachidonic acid into inflammation and pain-promoting PGE2. This sequence is illustrated in the bottom left side of Figure 1.

Anyone who is taking anti-inflammatory drugs, like ibuprofen, are doing so to inhibit the COX enzyme to block the production of pain-promoting PGE2. Table 2 lists some of the side effects of the medications used to inhibit PLA2, COX (prostaglandin E2), and the various pro-inflammatory cytokines. This is not a complete list, so if you are interested you can do an internet search for the individual medications. The website rxlist.com is a pharmacy website that provides reliable information.

Table 2 - Medications that inhibit inflammatory chemicals

Inflammatory chemicals	Medications	Side-effects
PLA2 (Phospholipase A2)	Corticosteroids (Prednisone, Celestone, Medrol, etc.)	Osteoporosis, hypertension, diabetes, weight gain, increased risk of infections
PGE2 (Prostaglandin E2)	COX inhibiting drugs: aspirin, ibuprofen (Advil), naproxen (Alleve), etc., and Celebrex, and Tylenol	Heartburn, stomach ulcers, high blood pressure, tinnitus, reduced bone healing
IL-1 (interleukin-1)	Kineret	Nausea, vomiting, diarrhea, stomach pain, joint pain, flu symptoms
IL-6 (interleukin-6)	Actemra	Sinus pain, sore throat, headache, dizziness, itching, urinary tract infection
IL-17 (interleukin-17)	Siliq, Taltz, Cosentyx	Joint pain, headache, fatigue, diarrhea, nausea, muscle pain
TNF (Tumor necrosis factor)	Enbrel, Remicade, Humira	Mild nausea, vomiting, diarrhea, headache, stomach pain, heart burn

Also, it is important to understand that these side effects typically occur with long-term use, which can vary from patient to patient. Please consult with your prescribing physician if you have any concerns about these medications, particularly if you have any of these side effects which can be disruptive to life in general, and also quite disruptive to you being able to engage in your favorite physical activities. It is much better to do everything we can to become free of the "flame" so that we do not end up taking these medications.

Please note that COX inhibiting drugs are typically called non-steroidal anti-inflammatory drugs (NSAIDs). Tylenol is not typically referred to as an NSAID; however, it also functions to inhibit the

COX enzyme to reduce the production of painful PGE2. The most common side-effect concern for Tylenol is liver damage, which has the potential to lead to liver failure if Tylenol is regularly taken by people who drink alcohol.

Back to Figure 1. The first thing that might catch your eye in Figure 1 is the cell in the top left with 666 in the cell membrane. The obvious Biblical reference notwithstanding, the 666 in this case refers to the overconsumption of omega-6 fatty acids that get inserted into cell membranes to create a pro-inflammatory state. We are supposed to consume a diet of less than a 4 to 1 ratio of omega-6 to omega-3 fatty acids in the diet, which is described in more detail in several chapters in *The DeFlame Diet* book (Chapters 18, 25, 26).

To the point of this chapter, an excess of omega-6 oil consumption promotes a state of free radical excess (7) and an over production of PGE2. Ideally, the ratio of omega-6 to omega-3 should be 1:1; which would lead to a 6363 configuration in the cell membrane. This represents an anti-free radical and anti-inflammatory state.

To the right of the cell is a blown-up image of a single phospholipid. An almost countless number of phospholipids are connected to make up the cell membrane of all cells in the human body. The circle represents what is called the phosphate head and the two vertical lines are fatty acids. It is important to understand that these fatty acids can be omega-6 or omega-3.

The last thing we want is to load up our cell membrane phospholipids with omega-6 fatty acids at the expense of omega-3 fatty acids. The average American eats a 10:1 to 25:1 ratio of omega-6 to omega-3, which is the result of fatty grain-fed animals and foods cooked/prepared with refined omega-6 oils from corn, sunflower, safflower, cottonseed, peanut, and soybean.

The proper omega-6 to omega-3 ratio should be less than 4:1 at worst; ideally as stated above, the ratio should be 1:1. In short, if you overeat omega-6 fatty acids, you will flame up all the cells in your body, including immune cells, which is the last thing we need if we get injured or exposed to a virus like SARS-CoV-2.

To the far right in Figure 1, it states that we need proper blood glucose levels to promote a proper free radical and antioxidant balance. Too much glucose in the blood supply leads to an excess production of free radicals, which cannot be controlled by dietary antioxidants or our body's antioxidant system.

Our antioxidant system involves both nutrients from our diet and our built-in antioxidant system that involves enzymes (which are a type of protein) that are a normal part of body function. In actual fact, nutrients and enzymes work together to keep free radical production at a healthy level.

The problem that most people have when it comes to understanding antioxidants and free radicals is that they do not understand that supplementation cannot fix the antioxidant enzyme system. In other words, overeating refined sugar, flour, and omega-6 oils creates a perpetual free radical state; in part by nutrient deficiency, but also by altering the normal function of our antioxidant enzyme system that favors an excess of free radicals.

This means that the most important antioxidant activity we can engage in is the elimination of excess calories from refined sugar, flour, and oils. Consider also that overeating these calories leads to obesity and type 2 diabetes, both of which are associated with an excess production of free radicals (8-10), which goes on 24 hours per day in an unrelenting fashion if one is obese and diabetic.

It is important to understand that overeating refined sugar, flour, and omega-6 oils creates a state wherein free radicals are perpetually overproduced, which cannot be corrected by supplements. This means we must DeFlame the diet to properly control free radical activity.

It is important to understand that free radicals are created constantly in the body by virtue of our dependency on oxygen to survive. Imagine that you bite an apple and let it sit on your counter. Within a short period of time, the flesh exposed to the air by the bite will begin to turn brown. This apple would rapidly rot compared to the one sitting next to it on the counter that was not bitten.

The apple browning process is called oxidation, and in the human body, such oxidation refers to free radical production. If you were to take two bites on opposite sides of the apple and squeeze lemon juice on one side, you will notice that it oxidizes much slower compared to the other side. This is because lemons contain antioxidants that prevent oxidation. Our goal with diet and supplements is the same as what the lemon is doing: to keep free radical production at a normal level to prevent chronic inflammation.

On the far left in Figure 1, you can see that a superoxide free radical (O_2-) is created and attacks a fatty acid in the cell membrane to create a lipid radical (R•), which can be converted into a lipid peroxyl radical (ROO•) [remember that lipid is synonymous with fat]. Both of these free radicals can stimulate NF-kB (a key inflammation signaling molecule) to stimulate ongoing inflammation, which manifests as an overproduction of PGE2 and pro-inflammatory cytokines. Notice that Zn (zinc) is next to O_2- and NF-kB to indicate that zinc is inhibitory to each of them. Such inhibition will lead to less cytokine production, as discussed earlier in this chapter in the context of the zinc supplementation study that reduced infections in older adults.

To the immediate right of the lipid peroxyl radical (ROO•) you can see vitamins E and C, which are specific nutrients that can reduce lipid and lipid peroxyl radicals. This is the extent to which most people think about free radicals and antioxidants, which is a very limited view.

Notice what happens to Vitamin E after it reduces the lipid peroxyl radical. Vitamin E now becomes a free radical. Vitamin C then comes along and reduces the vitamin E radical. But now vitamin C becomes a free radical. For context, adding supplemental vitamins E and C to an obese and hyperglycemic body does little if any good. Such chronically inflamed bodies lack the antioxidant wherewithal to reduce free radical E and C, which means that radicalized E and C participate in the inflammatory process. For radicalized E and C to be reduced, a substance called reduced glutathione (2GSH) must come to the rescue, which involves both nutrients and enzymes.

As stated above and in Table 1, 2GSH is called reduced glutathione, which is a special antioxidant that our bodies make from three amino acids called cysteine, glycine, and glutamic acid. The enzymes involved in the production of 2GSH are stimulated by a substance called Nrf2. There are many nutritional activators of Nrf2, such as vitamin D, lipoic acid, CoQ10, and polyphenols from ginger, turmeric, and most vegetation. Nrf2 activation is so important for body health that scientists published the following article:

> Lewis KN, et al. Nrf2, a guardian of healthspan and gatekeeper of species longevity. Integrative Comp Biol. 2010;50:829-43.

Notice in Figure 1 that reduced glutathione (2GSH) is utilized by the enzyme glutathione peroxidase, which requires selenium to reduce the vitamin C radical back to its normal antioxidant vitamin C. Not surprisingly, scientists identified that people in China with adequate selenium had better COVID-19 outcomes compared to those that were deficient (11). This is consistent with previous studies that have reported clinical benefits of selenium against viral and bacterial infections (12).

Notice that 2GSH is radicalized into GSSG• (oxidized glutathione) when it reduces vitamin C, which means that GSSG• must be reduced back into 2GSH. This requires the enzyme glutathione reductase (GR), which requires riboflavin (vitamin B2) and NADPH. Supplemental lipoic acid and CoQ10 can assist in the process of reducing GSSG• back into 2GSH. A recent scientific article suggests that a deficiency of reduced glutathione (2GSH) is a likely cause of serious manifestations and death in COVID-19 patients (13).

We need proper blood glucose levels to produce NADPH from NADP, which is why maintaining a proper blood glucose level is the most important thing we can do to keep free radical production in the normal range by reducing oxidized glutathione (GSSG•) back to reduced glutathione (GSH). There are two enzymes (GSPD and 6-GPD) involved in the production of NADPH, which require vitamin D to function properly. NADPH stands for nicotinamide adenine dinucleotide phosphate.

Nicotinamide, also referred to as niacinamide, is produced in the body from the B-vitamin niacin. As illustrated in Figure 1, niacinamide-containing NADP+ must be converted into niacinamide-containing NADPH, which is supported by vitamin D (14). We must produce adequate levels of NADPH in our bodies, as it is the key antioxidant that supports our body's entire antioxidant system.

Notice in Figure 1 that polyphenols and carotenoids in vegetables and fruit function as antioxidants to help keep vitamin E, vitamin C, and glutathione from becoming free radicalized. Polyphenols and carotenoids are the pigments that give vegetation their characteristic colors. Many people are aware that turmeric and ginger and other herbs/spices are anti-inflammatory and have antioxidant activity; it is the polyphenols in herbs/spices that are responsible for these beneficial functions. The fact that polyphenols support vitamins E, C, and glutathione demonstrates that no one should assume that all one needs to do is take supplements to insure normal antioxidant functions in the body.

Note also in Figure 1 that iodine protects fatty acids from being radicalized (15). This is a mostly unknown fact, which is why we should make sure to ingest adequate amounts of iodine or take an iodine supplement. Seaweed and fish are the best dietary sources of iodine. Supplemental iodine will be discussed in Chapter 13.

The end result of an excess of free radical generation is the overproduction of prostaglandin E2 (PGE2) and the proinflammatory cytokines as illustrated in the bottom left of Figure 1. When PGE2 and pro-inflammatory cytokines are overproduced during the majority of a lifespan, they participate in the gradual rotting or degradation of muscles, joints, tendons, spinal discs, bones, body fat, and arteries, which of course is a disaster for people who wish to remain physically active and quite characteristic of obese people with hyperglycemia.

The rotting process that occurs in each tissue is described in my recent book, *The DeFlame Diet to Stop Your Joints, Muscles, and Bones from Rotting*. As previously stated in this immune health book, these are the same people at the greatest risk for developing a severe case of COVID-19 and perhaps a catastrophic cytokine storm if infected by SARS-CoV-2.

Finally, let's consider a specific effect that excess free radical production has on immune cell function. Recall from Chapter 7 that macrophages and neutrophils are the two key immune cells that eliminate bacteria and viruses, as well as dead human cells and tissues from the body by phagocytosis, which is why these immune cells are also called phagocytes.

In the case of viruses, an infected cell will express a signaling molecule on its surface, which alerts phagocytes to eliminate the infected cell (16). We obviously do not want the capacity of immune cell phagocytosis to be impaired. Unfortunately, phagocytic activity is impaired in obese individuals (17) and those with type 2 diabetes (18).

Both obesity and diabetes are inflammatory pathological states associated with hyperglycemia and increased free radical production. Imagine an excess of glucose entering a macrophage, which causes this phagocyte to produce an excess of free radicals. This leads to a depressed ability of the phagocyte to engage in phagocytic activity (19).

To improve immune cell phagocytosis and viral removal, we should all endeavor to normalize the markers of inflammation discussed in Chapter 4. The most notable in the context of phagocytosis includes a normal body mass index (BMI) and waist/hip ratio for obesity, and fasting glucose, postprandial glucose, and hemoglobin A1c for hyperglycemia.

Supplements that have antioxidant functions also offer benefits. As stated above, this is because an excess production of free radicals by phagocytes reduces their phagocytic capacity (19). Thus, by reducing an excess of free radical production, antioxidant supplements are able to prevent this loss of phagocytic activity. The most studied in this regard is vitamin C (20). Zinc also appears to have a similar effect (21); however, we can broadly embrace the view that all antioxidant vitamins, minerals, and polyphenols have a similar effect.

In Chapter 13, I will discuss nutrient supplementation. Not surprisingly, my approach to supplementation is to focus on the key nutrients that have the biggest effect on helping control free radicals and inflammation, as opposed to picking supplements based on the name of a disease or condition. Trying to treat diseases with supplements tends to be inaccurate and unthorough, as the underlying body chemistry problems are often not properly addressed.

References

1. Read SA, Obeid S, Ahlenstiel C, Ahlenstiel G. The role of zinc in antiviral immunity. Adv Nutr. 2019;10:696-710.
2. Age-Related Eye Disease Study Research Group. A randomized, placebo-controlled clinical trial of high-dose supplementation with vitamins C and E, beta carotene, and zinc for age-related macular degeneration and vision loss. AREDS Report No. 8. Arch Opthalmol. 2001;119:1417-36.
3. Layana AG, Minnella AM, Garhofer G, et al. Vitamin D and age-related macular degeneration. Nutrients. 2017;9(10):1120.

4. Prasad AS, Beck FW, Bao B, et al. Zinc supplementation decreases incidence of infections in the elderly: effect of zinc on generation of cytokines and oxidative stress. Am J Clin Nutr. 2007;85:837-44.
5. Mariani E, Mangialasche F, Feliziani FT, et al. Effects of zinc supplementation on antioxidant enzyme activities in healthy old subjects. Exp Gerontology. 2008;43:445-51.
6. Prassad AS. Zinc in human health: effect of zinc on immune cells. Mol Med. 2008;14:353-57.
7. Berry EM. Are diets high in omega-6 polyunsaturated fatty acids unhealthy? Eur Heart J Suppl. 2001;3(Supplement D):D37-D41.
8. Hakkak R, Korourian S, Melnyk S. Obesity, oxidative stress and breast cancer risk. J Cancer Sci Ther. 2013;5(12):1000e129.
9. Kruk J. Overweight, obesity, oxidative stress and the risk of breast cancer. Asian Pac J Cancer Prev. 2014;15:9579-86.
10. Ullah A, Khan A, Khan I. Diabetes mellitus and oxidative stress—a concise review. Saudi Pharmaceutical J. 2016;24:547-553.
11. Zhang J, Taylor EW, Bennett K, et al. Association between regional selenium status and reported outcome of COVID-19 cases in China. Am J Clin Nutr. 2020;111:1297-99.
12. Steinbrenner H, Al-Quraishy S, Dkhil MA, Wunderlich F, Sies H. Dietary selenium in adjuvant therapy of viral and bacterial infections. Adv Nutr. 2015;6:73–82.
13. Polonikov A. Endogenous deficiency of glutathione as the most likely cause of serious manifestations and death in COVID-19 patients. Infectious diseases. 2020;6(7):1558-62.
14. Bao BY, Tin HJ, Hsu HJ, Lee YF. Protective role of 1-alpha, 25-dihydroxyvitamin D3 against oxidative stress in nonmalignant human prostate epithelial cells. Int J Cancer. 2008;122:2699-2706.
15. Venturi S, Venturi M. Iodine, PUFAs and iodolipids in health and diseases: an evolutionary perspective. Human Evolution. 2014;29:185-205.
16. Nainu F, Shiratsuchi A, Nakanishi Y. Induction of apoptosis and subsequent phagocytosis of virus-infected cells as an antiviral mechanism. Front Immunol. 2017;8: Article 1220.
17. Morais TC, Honorio-Franca AC, Fujimori M, et al. Melatonin action on the activity of phagocytes from the colostrum of obese women. Medicina. 2019;55:625.
18. Lecube A, Pachon G, Petriz J, Hernandez C, Simo R. Phagocytic activity is impaired in type 2 diabetes mellitus and increases after metabolic improvement. PLoS ONE. 2011;6(8):e23366.
19. Patel V, Dial K, Wu J, et al. Dietary antioxidants significantly attenuate hyperoxia-induced acute inflammatory lung injury by enhancing macrophage function via reducing the accumulation of airway HMGB1. Int J Molec Sci. 2020;21:977.
20. Carr AC, Maggini S. Vitamin C and immune function. Nutrients. 217;9:1211.

21. Gao H, Dai W, Zhao L, Min J, Wang F. The role of zinc and zinc homeostasis in macrophage function. J Immunol Res. 2018; Article ID: 6872621.

Chapter 12
Chronic gut inflammation and viral infection chemistry

Back in 2004, a paper was published in the Journal of the American Medical Association about small intestinal bacterial overgrowth (1), which is most commonly referred to by its acronym SIBO. Overgrowth of bacteria in the small intestine can lead to a host of symptoms, such as malaise, fatigue, depression, and widespread pain (1), which are the same symptoms people have when they are in bed with a cold or flu virus infection. Malaise and fatigue are also present in people infected with SARS-CoV-2 that are considered presymptomatic. In the context of SIBO, symptoms are caused by the absorption of a bacterial membrane component called bacterial endotoxin, which activates the immune system to uptick the level of prevailing body inflammation.

We have two main types of bacteria in the gut, half of which are gram-negative and the other half being gram-positive, which refers to how bacteria respond to a laboratory test called Gram staining. It is the gram-negative bacteria that have endotoxin in their cell walls. Figure 1 is an image of a gram-negative bacteria with an arrow pointing to endotoxin in the cell wall.

Figure 1

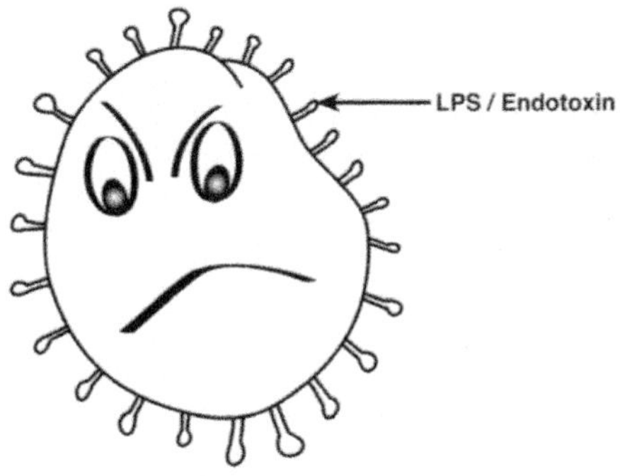

Bacterial endotoxin is also known as lipopolysaccharide or LPS for short. We begin to develop an endotoxin problem when we start to absorb an excess from the gut that leads to immune system activation. A way to understand how this works is to first appreciate that we humans have normally about as many bacterial cells in our bodies as we have human cells (2). But this changes when we overeat refined sugar, flour, and oils and consume too little dietary fiber.

Normally after we eat a meal, the food spends time being processed in the stomach before being sent to the small intestine where nutrients are absorbed. The digestive process involves both the absorption of nutrients and propulsion of non-absorbed material into the large intestine, where further processing occurs. Bacteria play an enormous food processing roll in the colon (large intestine) that ends in the production of fecal material that we release in a bowel movement. This is why half of the fecal dry mass is actually bacteria. Dry mass refers to fecal material when water is removed. The other half of the fecal dry mass is mostly fiber and undigested food residues.

The colon (large intestine) is adapted to house an enormous amount of bacteria, which is not the case for the small intestine. The purpose of the small intestine is nutrient extraction from food and then absorption of those nutrients. We do not want an excess of bacteria in the small intestine where nutrients are absorbed because this leads to the absorption of bacterial endotoxin, and this is what happens when we overeat refined sugar, flour, and oils and consume too little dietary fiber. Bacterial population of the small intestine starts to take on the appearance of the bacterial population of the large intestine as illustrated in Figure 2 on the next page.

Figure 2

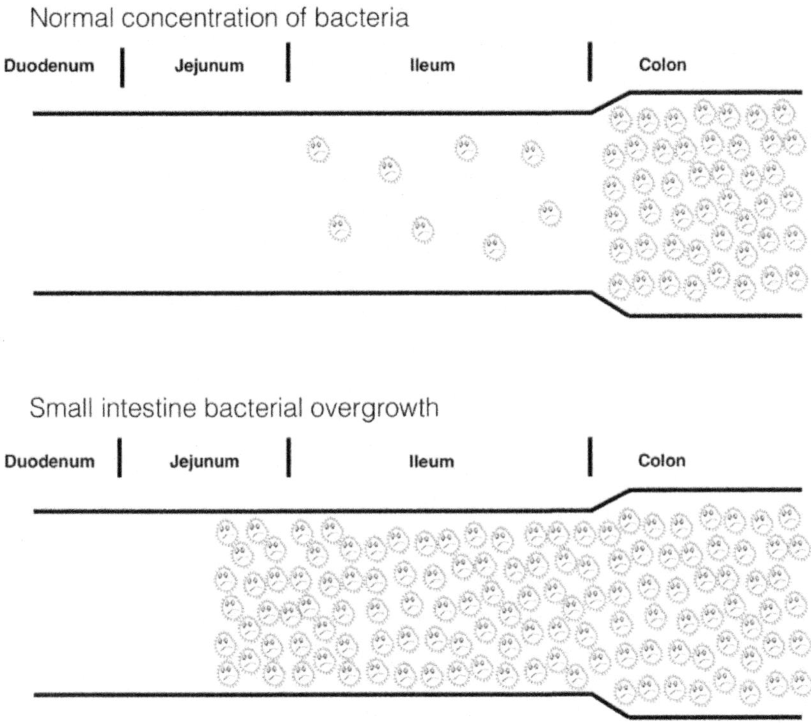

As stated earlier in this chapter, the overgrowth of bacteria in the small intestine can lead to a host of symptoms, such as malaise, fatigue, depression, and widespread pain, which is due to immune activation caused by the absorbed endotoxin released by gram-negative bacteria (1). This condition is more common in women than men, despite the fact that both women and men typically have the same pro-inflammatory diets. But because men generally eat more food mass than women, they are likely to get more dietary fiber, which is needed to propel food and bacteria from the small intestine to the large intestine.

The small intestine consists of the duodenum, jejunum, and ileum. The majority of nutrient absorption occurs in the duodenum and upper jejunum. As you might imagine, we do not just go to bed one night with normal bacteria in our small intestine and wake up the next day with overgrowth. It is important to understand that the overgrowth problem takes time to emerge and people respond differently with variable symptoms, so it is not readily diagnosable in the early stages. However, once a threshold of overgrowth is achieved, a common obvious symptom emerges, which is called postprandial bloating.

Bacterial fermentation of carbohydrates produces gases, such as hydrogen, carbon dioxide, and methane (3). When carbohydrates are eaten and delivered to the bacteria-infested small intestine, the gas that is produced causes the abdomen to bloat. This can be so severe that some women take on the appearance of being pregnant. Whether mild or severe, the person notices it within one hour of eating. For more information about this problem, my suggestion is to read the SIBO and gluten chapters in *The DeFlame Diet* book.

If one does not obviously bloat after eating carbohydrates, this does not mean that there is not a gut-derived endotoxin problem. There are essentially three stages by which circulating endotoxin levels rise, which I describe in *The DeFlame Diet* book:

> First, when we overeat refined sugar, flour, and oil calories, there is a greater release of endotoxin from the bacterial cell wall in our digestive tract, which is then absorbed into body circulation. This happens no matter if you are healthy or sick.
>
> Second, as people continue to overeat pro-inflammatory calories, the digestive tract flames up and becomes more permeable, which allows for a greater amount of endotoxin to enter body circulation.
>
> Third, as body fat accumulates, people become obese and develop the pro-inflammatory metabolic syndrome. The metabolic syndrome is a pro-inflammatory state that includes the transformation of healthy HDL and LDL into pro-inflammatory HDL and LDL. This is problematic

> because it is healthy HDL and LDL that trap, process, and eliminate excess endotoxin. When this happens, the inflamed LDL and HDL can no longer properly process and eliminate endotoxin.

In the absence of post-prandial bloating, there are several surrogate markers that correlate to circulating endotoxin levels, such as waist circumference, waist/hip ratio, triglycerides, and hemoglobin A1c (4,5). This is why understanding Chapter 4 in this book is so important. When we normalize the inflammatory markers, this has a broad, full-body DeFlaming effect.

Psychosocial stressors can also increase circulating endotoxin levels (6,7). This is because such stressors create a hyperpermeable state within the small intestine. In common language, people refer to this as leaky gut syndrome. Normally, the small intestine is not permeable, or just minimally permeable, to immune-stimulating food particles or bacterial antigens like endotoxin, but this changes for stressed-out people.

The stress response involves the production of fight-or-flight chemicals. The most notable are cortisol and adrenaline (more commonly called epinephrine). Another chemical produced when we are stressed-out is called noradrenaline, which is more commonly known as norepinephrine. Certain types of nerve endings release norepinephrine and when this happens in the gut it becomes hyperpermeable (7), as illustrated in Figure 3 on the next page.

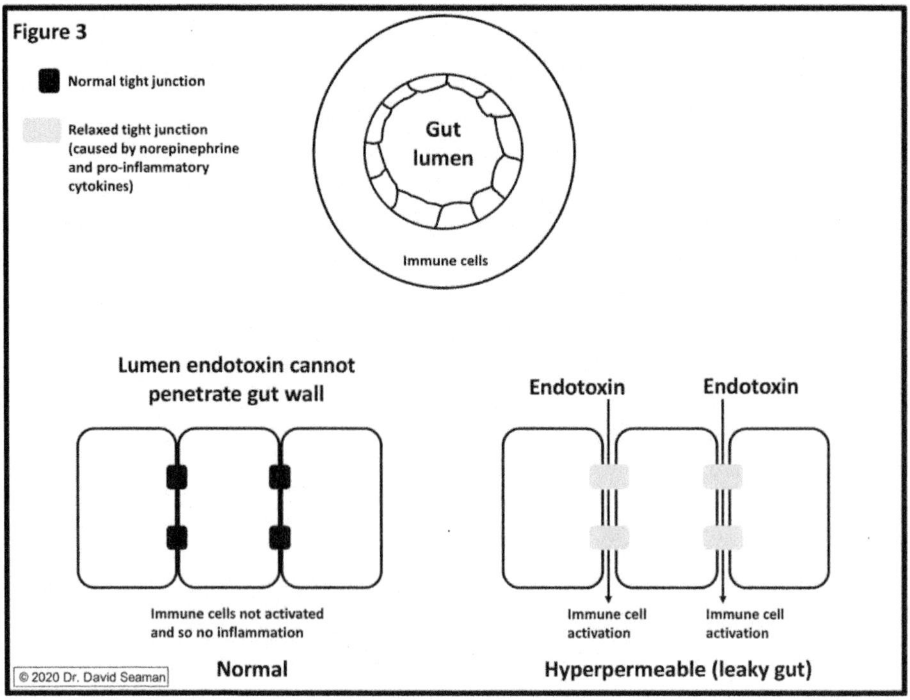

The small intestine lumen, or gut lumen, refers to the space where food is digested and then absorbed. The lumen also contains trillions of bacteria. Tight junctions bind together gut cells called enterocytes, which prevents undigested food particles, bacteria, and endotoxin from being absorbed. Beneath the layer of enterocytes are immune cells that are there in case such substances get past the enterocytes.

Both pro-inflammatory cytokines and the norepinephrine released as part of the stress response causes tight junctions to become relaxed. This leads to an excess absorption of endotoxin and other substances. When endotoxin is absorbed, it activates gut wall immune cells to produce more cytokines, which further relaxes the tight junctions to perpetuate the hyperpermeable state.

Elevated endotoxin levels have been correlated to many conditions, such as obesity, the metabolic syndrome, diabetes, atherosclerosis, and others, which I outlined in *The DeFlame Diet* book. Endotoxin levels can return to normal if people DeFlame their diets and become physically active. Endotoxin is never measured in clinical practice.

However, endotoxin levels are measured in the research setting and are known to correlate with other inflammatory markers, as mentioned earlier in this chapter. So, if you normalize all the inflammatory markers discussed in Chapter 4, endotoxin levels typically normalize as well.

Several key nutrients also support normal gut barrier integrity to prevent hyperpermeability, those being magnesium, vitamin D, omega-3 fatty acids, polyphenols, and probiotics (8-18). Following The DeFlame Diet and taking these supplements provides us with the best way to create a DeFlamed state in the gut and the rest of the body.

A final comment on the maintenance of proper gut barrier integrity. Gluten-free diets are still very popular and they are most relevant for people with celiac disease and gluten sensitivity. One of the effects that gluten has in the gut is to compromise tight junctions to promote hyperpermeability and chronic inflammation (19). The degree to which this happens in non-celiac and non-gluten sensitivity patients is not known; however, most people would do well to go gluten-free for a week to a month to identify if they are reactive. Gluten is discussed in more detail in its own chapter in *The DeFlame Diet* book.

References

1. Lin HC. Small intestinal bacterial overgrowth: a framework for understanding irritable bowel syndrome. JAMA. 2004;292:852-58
2. Sender R, Fuchs S, Milo R. Are we really vastly outnumbered? Revisiting the ratio of bacterial to host cells in humans. Cell. 2016;164:337-40.
3. Scaldaferri F, Nardone O, Lopetuso LR, et al. Intestinal gas production and gastrointestinal symptoms: from pathogenesis to clinical implication. Eur Rev Med Pharm Sciences. 2013;17(Suppl 2):2-110.
4. Miller MA, McTernan PG, Hart AL, et al. Ethnic and sex differences in circulating endotoxin levels: A novel marker of atherosclerotic and cardiovascular risk in a British multi-ethnic population. Atherosclerosis. 2009;203(2):494-502.
5. Troseid M, Nestvold TK, Rudi K, et al. Plasma lipopolysaccharide is closely associated with glycemic control and abdominal obesity: evidence from bariatric surgery. Diabetes Care. 2013;36(11):3627-3632.
6. Peirce JM, Alvina K. The role of inflammation and the gut microbiome in depression and anxiety. J Neuro Res. 2019;97:1223-41.

7. de Punder K, Pruimboom L. Stress induces endotoxemia and low-grade inflammation by increasing barrier permeability. Front Immunol. 2015;6:223.
8. Weglicki WB, Mak IT, Chmielinska JJ, et al. The role of magnesium deficiency in cardiovascular and intestinal inflammation. Mag Res. 2010;23:S199-206.
9. Pachikian BD, Neyrinck AM, Deldicque L, et al. Changes in intestinal Bifidobacteria levels are associated with the inflammatory response in magnesium-deficiency mice. J Nutr. 2010;140:509-14.
10. Tabbaa M, Golubic M, Roizen MF, Bernstein AM. Docosahexaenoic acid, inflammation, and bacterial dysbiosis in relation to periodontal disease, inflammatory bowel disease, and the metabolic syndrome. Nutrients. 2013;5:3299-3310.
11. Campbell EL, MacManus CF, Kominsky DJ, et al. Resolvin E1-induced intestinal alkaline phosphatase promotes resolution of inflammation through LPS detoxification. PNAS. 2010;107:14298-303.
12. Kong J, Zhang Z, Musch MW, et al. Novel role of the vitamin D receptor in maintaining integrity of the intestinal mucosal barrier. Am J Physiol Gastrointest Liver Physiol. 2008;294:G208-16.
13. Sun J. Vitamin D and mucosal immune function. Curr Opin Gastroenterol. 2010;26:591-95.
14. Zhang Y, Wu S, Lu R, et al. Tight junction *CLDN2* gene is a direct target of the vitamin D receptor. Sci Reports. 2015;5:10642.
15. Shimizu M. Multifunctions of dietary polyphenols in the regulation of intestinal inflammation. J Food Drug Analysis. 2017;25:93-99.
16. Bernardi S, Del Bo C, Marino M, et al. Polyphenols and intestinal permeability: rationale and future perspectives. J Agric Food Chem. 2020;68:1816-29.
17. Sherman PM, Ossa JC, Johnson-Henry K. Unraveling mechanisms of action of probiotics. Nutr Clin Pract. 2009;24:10-14.
18. Sartor RB. Bacteria in Crohn's Disease: Mechanisms of Inflammation and Therapeutic Implications. J Clin Gastroenterol. 2007; 41(Suppl 1):S37-S43.
19. Fasano A. Zonulin and its regulation of intesti- nal barrier function: the biological door to inflammation, autoimmunity, and cancer. *Physiol Rev*. 2011;91(1):151-175.

Chapter 13
Supplements for immune health

In several chapters in this book, various nutritional supplements are discussed. It is quite common for people to misunderstand the purpose of nutritional supplements. They are typically viewed in the context of taking medications, which is not the proper way to view nutritional supplements. The next few paragraphs describe what I mean.

A pro-inflammatory lifestyle, which includes a poor diet, stress, lack of sleep, and sedentary living, cause our bodies to flame up and then express chronic pain, depression, chronic diseases (heart disease, cancer, etc.), and have worse outcomes when infected by a virus like SARS-CoV-2.

Approximately 70% of the US population is overweight or obese, which represents a state of chronic inflammation due to the overconsumption of refined sugar, flour, and omega-6 oils. It is important to understand that the overconsumption of refined food calories and not eating enough vegetation will eventually lead to deficiencies of the key nutrients listed in Figure 1 on the next page. When this diet-induced pro-inflammatory state manifests, no drug or combination of drugs can remotely restore a normal state of non-inflammatory chemistry to the body.

The same holds true for supplements, which is why it is so important to achieve and maintain a body weight that allows for the markers of inflammation outlined in Chapter 4 to return to normal. In most cases, when the markers of inflammation are normal, people can live most of their lives without medications and be free of chronic diseases. However, this does not necessarily mean we should avoid taking key supplements.

Many people believe that if you eat properly, you do not need to take any supplements. I disagree with this view. My perspective is that we should all take certain supplements, those being magnesium, iodine, omega-3 fatty acids, polyphenols, vitamin D, vitamin C, and zinc. All of these nutrients, save for magnesium, are included in Figure 1, which was also used in Chapter 11 about free radicals and antioxidants. The reason for showing you the image again is to reinforce that we should be taking supplements for the purpose of reducing free radicals and chronic inflammation, which are the foundational causes of health problems as made plainly clear for many years in standard pathology books (1).

If you try to take supplements to "treat" conditions and diseases, you will find that many of the same supplements are recommended for different conditions, such as vitamin D, omega-3 fatty acids, ginger/turmeric, vitamin C, zinc, and CoQ10. The reason for this is because these overlapping supplements are the ones that are anti-inflammatory, which means that our dietary and supplementation focus should be on reducing chronic inflammation. This also means that the title of this current chapter is not technically correct, as every supplement discussed in this chapter is also good for joint health, muscle health, heart health, brain health, mental health, etc.

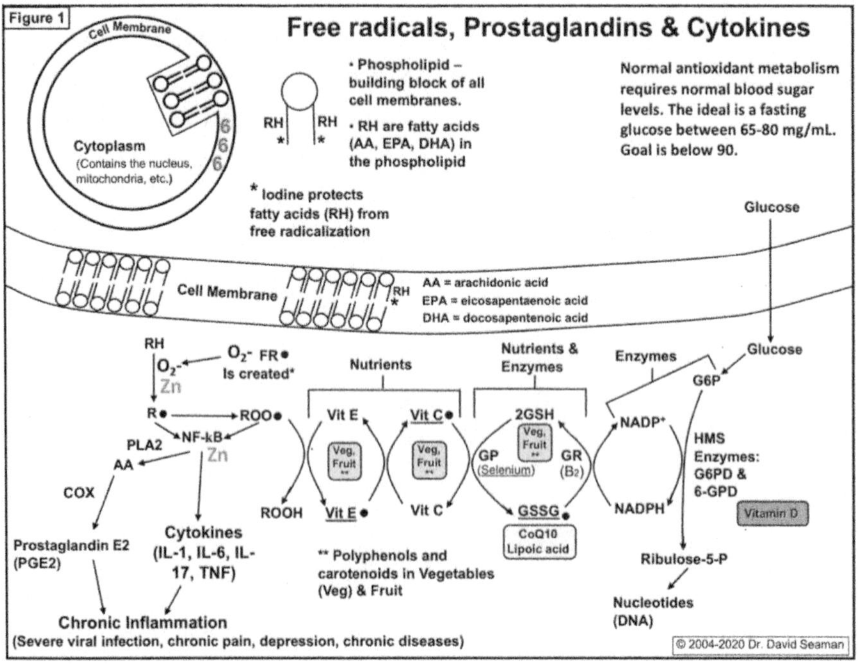

Without the key nutrients in Figure 1, free radicals and inflammation would run wild and lead to the expression of chronic pain, depression, and other chronic diseases, and make one more susceptible to severe viral infections. Again, this is why I focus on reducing free radicals and chronic inflammation as opposed to trying to "treat" specific diseases, since they are all caused by the same underlying pro-inflammatory state.

With the above in mind, we can use Figure 1 to focus on immune health. Recall in Chapter 7 that I discussed the topic of phagocytosis, which is how immune cells rid the body of tissue debris after injury, bacteria, and virus-infected cells. Recall that phagocytosis is impaired in obese individuals (2) and those with type 2 diabetes (3).

Recall also that an excess production of free radicals by immune cells reduces their phagocytic capacity (4). By reducing an excess of free radical production, antioxidant supplements are able to help prevent this loss of phagocytic activity. The most studied in this regard are vitamin C and zinc (5,6), which is why they are always discussed in the context of immune health. However, you should understand that any supplement that has antioxidant activities will have a similar benefit. You should also understand that by reducing excess free radical activity, there is a commensurate reduction of inflammatory activity.

I personally take all of the following supplements at the amounts described below. I don't take all of them all the time and I have no specific rhyme or reason for when I cycle on and off. It just seems to happen. The only one I absolutely take every day is magnesium, which I discuss below.

All of the following supplements are nutrients found in foods, so there are rarely contraindications. For people taking medications, there may be contraindications, so you should consult with your prescribing physician. The main medication of concern is Coumadin, also known as warfarin, which is a powerful blood thinner. This is because the anti-inflammatory effect of most supplements will augment the blood thinning effect of Coumadin.

Magnesium

Magnesium is not included in Figure 1; however it is known that deficiencies increase free radical production (7). Here is why I absolutely always take magnesium. There are more than 300 metabolic reactions in the body that require magnesium, and many involve anti-inflammatory actions (8). The typical recommendation for magnesium supplementation is 400-1000 mg per day. I personally take at least 1000 mg per day. I often take more if I am feeling especially stressed out because stress physiology depletes body magnesium (8).

In the context of COVID-19, researchers in Singapore supplemented older subjects with magnesium (150 mg), vitamin D (1000 IU), and vitamin B12 (500 mcg) (9). Only 17.6% of supplemented patients required oxygen therapy, while 61.5% who did not receive supplements required oxygen.

Iodine

Iodine is most known for its relationship to the production of thyroid hormones. Not well known is what was described in Chapter 11 about iodine; that it functions as an antioxidant and protects cell membrane fatty acids from free radical attack. This is important for all cell membranes. However, in the context of disease risk, it is especially important for protection against breast cancer and prostate cancer (10,11).

The Japanese population consumes between 1000-3000 micrograms (mcg) per day (10), which is derived largely from seaweed and much less from fish. It turns out that seaweed and fish are natural sources of both omega-3 fatty acids and iodine, which is one of the reasons why a traditional Japanese diet is so healthy and associated with minimal disease risk. When Japanese people move to the United States and adopt a pro-inflammatory American diet, they begin to express the same chronic diseases as Americans.

In the United States, the upper limit recommendation for iodine is only 1100 mcg per day. I personally take 1000 mcg per day in addition to my diet, which means I choose to ingest iodine based on the Japanese intake pattern. As far as I can tell, the 1000-3000 mcg level is likely to be a problem for only people with hypothyroidism caused by Hashimoto's disease (3). Many people with Hashimoto's disease cannot take any iodine. If you consider taking iodine, consult with your physician if you have concerns about hypothyroidism caused by Hashimoto's disease.

Omega-3 fatty acids

Supplementing with omega-3 fatty acids from fish oil is quite common and many people do it. The typical recommendation is to take between 1000-3000 milligrams (mg) per day. The purpose of taking omega-3 fatty acids is to create a proper balance of omega-6 to omega-3 fatty acids in our cell membranes, which was discussed in the previous chapter. Recall that most Americans consume a 10:1 to 25:1 ratio of omega-6 to omega-3 fatty acids, which loads up cell membranes with omega-6 fatty acids as reflected by the 666 in Figure 1.

There are two mistakes that people make when they supplement with omega-3 fish oil. The first mistake most people make is to take omega-3 fish oil supplements without simultaneously eliminating the excess omega-6 oils. As stated previously, omega-6 fatty acids are found in great abundance in oils from corn, safflower, sunflower, cottonseed, peanut, and soybean oils. The most notable caloric culprits that are rich in omega-6 fatty acids include cakes, desserts, donuts, French fries (and other deep-fried foods), and oil roasted nuts. Additionally, all feed lot-raised animals (meat, fish, chicken) have an abundance of omega-6 fatty acids compared to their natural counterparts. This is a consequence of the excess omega-6 fatty acids in the feed they consume.

The second mistake is to not recognize that omega-3 rich foods in nature are also the best sources of omega-3 fatty acid-protecting iodine. Seaweed is particularly abundant, while fish is less and fish oil contains virtually no iodine due to the distillation process involved in making fish oil supplements.

As my knowledge about iodine has expanded, I now believe it is unwise to take omega-3 fish oil supplements without also ensuring adequate iodine intake as outlined in the previous section about iodine.

Polyphenols

As described in Chapter 11, polyphenols and carotenoids are found in vegetation. I never supplement with carotenoids because I eat lots of green vegetables, which are a rich source. I do supplement ginger and/or turmeric to increase my intake of polyphenols. I also often get polyphenols derived from lemons. The typical recommendation is about 1000-2000 milligrams per day of supplemental polyphenols. When I make fresh vegetable juice, I always use ginger and/or turmeric as well as lemons and/or limes. We also derive anti-inflammatory polyphenols from coffee and tea, so both of these beverages should be viewed as anti-inflammatory.

Vitamin D

The details about vitamin D were discussed in Chapter 10. Recall that in the context of immune health, a deficiency in vitamin D leads to an immune cell profile that resembles that of a viral infection. Recall also from Chapter 10 that vitamin D dosing should be based on our vitamin D level in the blood. I typically take about 5000-10,000 IUs per day. Remember also from Chapter 10 that vitamin D is required for immune cells to make anti-microbial peptides called cathelicidins and defensins.

Zinc

Recall from the beginning of Chapter 11 about free radicals and antioxidants that a zinc supplementation study was described. A total of fifty subjects (aged 55-87) took either 45 mg of zinc per day or a placebo for one year. The study was double-blind and placebo-controlled, which means that the subjects and scientists did not know which 25 subjects received zinc and which 25 subjects received the placebo. At the end of the year study period, it was determined that only 29% of subjects taking zinc had infections, while 88% of those taking the placebo had infections. The reason for this is because those taking the zinc had significantly reduced oxidative stress and pro-inflammatory cytokines (12), which made them significantly less likely to have an acute phase response to viruses and other stressors during that one-year period.

I do not know if anyone knows for sure how much zinc one should take on a daily basis. The recommended daily allowance (RDA) of zinc is about 10 mg per day for adults. With this mind, we also know from the zinc study discussed above that supplementing with 45 mg of zinc per day for a year was beneficial and no one suffered with side-effects, which means that we can tolerate a zinc level well above the RDA. My suspicion is that taking 20-30 mg of zinc per day is reasonable. I think this applies to most people, as regular vigorous exercise and stress can deplete the body of zinc (13). This actually applies to most nutrients, as the RDAs typically do not take into consideration chronic stress and the stress of exercise.

Vitamin C

We now know that vitamin C levels in white blood cells are over ten times higher than blood levels, which may indicate functional roles of the vitamin in these immune system cells (14). So, it is not surprising that since the 1970s, vitamin C supplementation has been recommended for treating and preventing colds. In 1993, scientists published the results of study that tracked upper respiratory tract infections in ultramarathon runners. In a double-blind trial, 46 athletes received 600 mg of supplemental vitamin C for 21 days prior to the marathon, while another 46 took a placebo (15). A total of 33% in the supplemented group reported infections, while infections were reported in 68% of those taking the placebo.

A recent review article suggests that the cold-preventing effect of vitamin C is possible; however, large doses are required, which are higher than most people would think. "Two controlled trials found a statistically significant dose–response, for the duration of common cold symptoms, with up to 6-8 grams/day of vitamin C. Thus, the negative findings of some therapeutic common cold studies might be explained by the low doses of 3-4 grams/day of vitamin C." (14) These and other details related to vitamin C supplementation and colds is too much to discuss in this book. If this topic is an interest of yours, you should get and read this free article by doing an internet search for, "Hemila vitamin C and infections," and you will get this paper:

Hemila H. Vitamin C and infections. Nutrients. 2017;9:339.

From my perspective, I do not look at vitamin C supplementation in the context of cold prevention because it is very common for people to not take vitamin C and still not suffer from colds or the flu. Not surprisingly, I think it is about controlling chronic inflammation and being resilient to acute inflammatory challenges, the most notable being physical exhaustion, sleep deprivation, and severe mental/emotional stressors. Several articles have discussed the importance of vitamin C in the context of dealing with stressors (16-18). The dosing amount that seems adequate for this purpose and for supporting immune function is 1000-3000 mg per day.

Additional supplements

I also take coenzyme Q10 (100 mg/day), which has three key functions. It supports ATP synthesis, which is what the body uses for cellular energy, it is an important antioxidant, and it has anti-inflammatory functions.

I also take probiotics in a randomly cyclical fashion. Probiotics have three domains of activity, the first being in the gut lumen where they interact and DeFlame other bacteria. Probiotics also interact with enterocytes to help support tight junctions to prevent a hyperpermeable gut. Finally, probiotics help to DeFlame immune activity in the gut wall. I discuss probiotics in more detail in the probiotic chapter in *The DeFlame Diet* book.

References

1. Cotran RS, Kumar V, Collins T. Robbins' Pathologic Basis of Disease. 6th ed. Philadelphia: WB Saunders; 1999: p.1-112
2. Morais TC, Honorio-Franca AC, Fujimori M, et al. Melatonin action on the activity of phagocytes from the colostrum of obese women. Medicina. 2019;55:625.
3. Lecube A, Pachon G, Petriz J, Hernandez C, Simo R. Phagocytic activity is impaired in type 2 diabetes mellitus and increases after metabolic improvement. PLoS ONE. 2011;6(8):e23366.
4. Patel V, Dial K, Wu J, et al. Dietary antioxidants significantly attenuate hyperoxia-induced acute inflammatory lung injury by enhancing macrophage function via reducing the accumulation of airway HMGB1. Int J Molec Sci. 2020;21:977.
5. Carr AC, Maggini S. Vitamin C and immune function. Nutrients. 217;9:1211.
6. Gao H, Dai W, Zhao L, Min J, Wang F. The role of zinc and zinc homeostasis in macrophage function. J Immunol Res. 2018; Article ID: 6872621.
7. Zheltova AA, Kharitonova MV, Iezhitsa IN, Spasov AA. Magnesium deficiency and oxidative stress: an update. Biomedicine. 2016;6:8-14.
8. Seaman DR. The DeFlame Diet: deflame your diet, body, and mind. Wilmington; Shadow Panther Press. 2016.
9. Tan CW, Ho LP, Kalimuddin S, et al. A cohort study to evaluate the effect of combination vitamin D, magnesium and vitamin B12 (DMB) on progression to severe outcome in older COVID-19 patients. medRxivf. June 10, 2020. doi: https://doi.org/10.1101/2020.06.01.20112334
10. Seaman DR. The DeFlame Diet for Breast Health and Cancer Prevention. Wilmington; Shadow Panther Press. 2019.
11. Venturi S, Venturi M. Iodine, PUFAs and iodolipids in health and diseases: an evolutionary perspective. 2014;29:185-205.
12. Prasad AS, Beck FW, Bao B, et al. Zinc supplementation decreases incidence of infections in the elderly: effect of zinc on generation of cytokines and oxidative stress. Am J Clin Nutr. 2007;85:837-44.
13. Cordova A, Navas FJ. Effect of training on zinc metabolism: changes in serum and sweat zinc concentrations in sportsmen. Nutr Metab. 1998;42:274-82.
14. Hemila H. Vitamin C and infections. Nutrients. 2017;9:339.
15. Peters EM, Goetzsche JM, Grobbelaar B, Noakes TD. Vitamin C supplementation reduces the incidence of postrace symptoms of upper-respiratory-tract infection in ultramarathon runners. Am J Clin Nutr. 1993;57:170-74.
16. Hooper MH, Carr A, Marik PE. The adrenal-vitamin C axis: from fish to guinea pigs and primates. 2019;23(1):29.
17. Marik PE. Vitamin C: an essential "stress hormone" during sepsis. J Thoracic Dis. 2020;12(suppl 1):S84-S88.
18. Brody S, Preut R, Schommer K, Schurmeyer TH. A randomized controlled trial of high dose ascorbic acid for reduction of blood pressure, cortisol, and subjective responses to psychological stress. Psychopharmacol. 2002;159:319-324.

Chapter 14
Bioweapons, exosomes, 5G technology, and COVID-19 facts and fiction

Introduction

By the time you have reached this chapter, you should understand that COVID-19 is health crisis and NOT a virus crisis. Unfortunately, governments have absolutely embraced it as a virus crisis and not a health crisis. This is why economies were locked down and many officials have claimed that we all need to be vaccinated before society and the economy can move back to normal.

I think the notion that we cannot get back to normal until there is a coronavirus vaccine is completely ridiculous. Again, COVID-19 is a health/obesity crisis and NOT a virus crisis or lack-of-a-vaccine crisis. From this perspective, it does not really matter if we are dealing with a legit virus, a bioweapon, pro-inflammatory exosomes, or 5G radiation. This is because, save for the rare outlier, only sick and unhealthy people are suffering from severe cases of COVID-19.

Why do some people focus on bioweapons, exosomes, and 5G technology? I think it is because people have been conditioned by government actions to distrust government, especially when these actions appear authoritarian in nature. People justifiably perceive forced lockdowns, fines for going in the ocean, and mandatory SARS-CoV-2 vaccination as an authoritarian overreach, which is fueled by the fact that we have been told by the media, amidst their simultaneous fear mongering, that it is sick people with comorbidities who are at risk.

With the above in mind, you should understand that governments, and the people in power, rarely if ever confess to making a mistake because it would undermine their authority. They often engage in outright lies, which should not be a shock to anyone. For example, consider the fact that the Tonkin Gulf incident, which caused the United States to officially enter the Vietnam War, never happened.

The US alleged that North Vietnamese forces attacked two American naval destroyers (USS Maddox and USS Turner Joy) in the Tonkin Gulf. This led the US Congress to pass the Tonkin Gulf Resolution, which authorized President Johnson to send US troops into Vietnam. In short, the US involvement in the war led to the deaths of some 60,000 American soldiers who went to fight in Vietnam based on an event that NEVER happened. Hundreds of thousands of Vietnamese civilians were also killed during the war.

Fast forward to the Second Gulf War that began in 2003 during George W. Bush's presidential era. Two lies were perpetuated by the US government and its media outlets about Iraq, which were the evidence used to start the war. First, Colin Powell alleged that Iraq was well on its way to making weapons of mass destruction. In his presentation to the United Nations, Powell made the case that Saddam Hussein was stockpiling anthrax. Second, it was implied by the Bush crew that Saddam Hussein was involved in taking down the Twin Towers on 9/11 and that he was likely making nuclear weapons. Both were lies that led to hundreds of thousands of unnecessary deaths.

These are just two of many examples of how the US government overtly lied Americans into war, which led to massive casualties and societal suffering. There is also no shortage of lies that are told to us by politicians on a regular basis. Democrat voters point out the lies made by Republicans in office and Republican voters point out the lies made by Democrats in office. The point is that both parties regularly engage in lying and very few people would argue against the fact that our political system is corrupt. So no one should be surprised that many people do not trust what the government says about the coronavirus crisis.

My opinion is that we common people should send a clear message to congress indicating that it is very clear to us that they are gravely mistaken about the fanciful notion that COVID-19 is a virus crisis or lack-of-a-vaccine crisis. Congress and state governors should confess that they erred in their assumptions about SARS-CoV-2. Most should probably resign.

COVID-19 is clearly a health crisis, just as diabetes, heart disease, cancer, Alzheimer's disease, depression, chronic pain, and other chronic conditions are also health crises. And even if COVID-19 is caused by a bioweapon, exosomes, or 5G technology, it is still a health crisis, as only unhealthy people suffer with severe complications. In other words, our focus should be on DeFlaming ourselves into a state of health, so that we can withstand pro-inflammatory stressors, be they viral, mental/emotional, or physical.

With the above in mind, do bioweapons, exosomes, or 5G theories have any merit? I personally do not know the answer to this question, but my feeling is that they are quite unlikely. My view is that SARS-CoV-2 is a legit virus and that COVID-19, the disease that is caused by SARS-CoV-2, can be lethal for some. It is also my view that COVID-19 is being handled in a shameless fashion by government authorities who reject the truth that it is a health/obesity crisis and instead embrace the fantasy that it is a virus crisis and lack-of-a-vaccine crisis, which serves to fuel conspiratorial thinking.

Bioweapon theory

I suspect that SARS-CoV-2 is not bioweapon. However, we do absolutely know that bioweapons are real. Many countries have bioweapons research and manufacturing facilities, including the two countries with the biggest economies in the world, those being the United States and China.

We also know that the Wuhan Institute of Virology is located in Wuhan, China where the SARS-CoV-2 outbreak began. Additionally, we know that Dr. Anthony Fauci provided NIH funding to New York City-based EcoHealth Alliance that has had a longtime partnership with the Wuhan Institute of Virology. Together they work on identifying unknown bat coronaviruses (1).

Coincidentally, in October 2019, the city of Wuhan hosted the 2019 Military World Games, which brought in almost 10,000 military athletes from over 140 countries. Then, just two months later in Wuhan, we were alerted by the Chinese authorities that SARS-CoV-2 had been identified. These coincidences naturally cause many people to question the legitimacy of the story that SARS-CoV-2 emerged from animals in the Wuhan wet market by mere coincidence.

Whether SARS-CoV-2 is a bioweapon or not, the fact remains that it only compromises excessively inflamed people. For this reason, it is very difficult for me to believe the bioweapon theory.

5G theory

To me, the 5G theory is pretty bizarre. I do not know enough about wireless technology to comment much on this theory other than to say that I think it is highly unlikely. It is difficult for me to believe that 5G radio waves are being used to spread the coronavirus that will then cause COVID-19 in obese diabetics and old frail people, as well as otherwise highly inflamed individuals.

About two weeks before this book was released, I became aware of an article entitled, "5G technology and induction of coronavirus in skin cells." It was published in the *Journal of Biological Regulators and Homeostatic Agents* on July 16, 2020 and withdrawn shortly thereafter. Even the abstract was withdrawn, which I managed to save a copy of before it was removed. Here are the first and last sentences of the abstract:

> "In this research, we show that 5G millimeter waves could be absorbed by dermatologic cells acting like antennas, transferred to other cells and play the main role in producing Coronaviruses in biological cells... Thus, 5G millimeter waves could be good candidates for applying in constructing virus-like structures such as Coronaviruses (COVID-19) within cells."

To me this does not mean that SARS-CoV-2 was caused by 5G and this is primarily because millions of people had 5G technology in their homes long before COVID-19 appeared on the scene. My position remains the same. SARS-CoV-2 only compromises the excessively inflamed among us, which means that if we were all healthy and DeFlamed, 5G-induction of SARS-CoV-2 would be mostly meaningless.

Exosome theory

The exosome theory suggests that viruses are really exosomes produced by a stressed body, which signal the immune system to pump out inflammatory chemicals to make us sick. Fueling this notion is the following statement from a 2003 article about HIV (2):

> "The virus is fully an exosome in every sense of the word."

If you read this 2003 article, it does NOT say that HIV is not a virus; rather it says that viruses hijack exosomes. Exosomes are vesicles produced by human cells that contain biologically active RNAs, lipids, and proteins, which are involved in cell to cell communication (3), making it a perfect vector for a virus. In other words, viruses are not exosomes. Scientists are even looking to see if they can use exosomes to inhibit viral infections (4).

Why COVID-19 is and IS NOT a scam-demic

The information discussed in this book should have made it very clear that COVID-19 is a very real condition for some people and absolutely nothing to worry about for the vast majority. In other words, the coronavirus is absolutely a scam-demic for some but NOT for others.

On May 18, 2020, Yahoo News published an article entitled, *He thought the coronavirus was 'a fake crisis.' Then he contracted it* (5). The story is about Brian Hitchens and links to his Facebook page which contains his comments. Here is the quote from the Yahoo article that contains a link to his Facebook page:

> In a lengthy post on May 12, Hitchens said that he was once among those who thought the coronavirus "is a fake crisis" that was "blown out of proportion" and "wasn't that serious."

If you look at Brian, you will notice that he is morbidly obese. The research is very clear about obesity and COVID-19 severity, such that obesity is a most significant risk factor as described previously in this book. All you need to do to verify this fact is to read this book and do an internet search for "obesity and COVID-19," and scientific and news media articles will appear. One article explains how obesity triples the odds of more severe symptoms with COVID-19 (6). This is likely because, as described in Chapter 9, the immune cell profile within the obese body resembles that of a viral infection, an absolute fact that is virtually unknown by most people.

The fact that Hitchens was unaware of this relationship between obesity and viral infection speaks mightily to the noise created by the government and news media. This means that the government, its media, and the medical industrial complex have completely failed Hitchens and his fellow morbidly obese Americans. And mostly what the lockdown has done is make people fatter and sicker, such that the term "Quarantine 15" is being used to describe the weight gain that is occurring for people during lockdown. You should know that such weight gain is almost always associated with high levels of blood glucose, which is exactly what drives COVID-19 severity as described earlier in this book.

In short, COVID-19 is very, very real and NOT a scam for obese people, especially when these people are hyperglycemic, hypertense, and suffering from heart disease. Hyperglycemia may be the biggest risk factor, as it facilitates the entry of the virus into lung cells (7) which is outlined in Chapter 2 of this book. This means that the government, its media, and medical profession should have used COVID-19 as a call to fitness for most Americans. Indeed, 70% of Americans are overweight or obese and this terrific opportunity to encourage health improvements has been totally ignored.

Consider how much television and print/online media has been devoted to COVID-19 and all we hear/read about is the dangerous virus and the need for a vaccine to return to normal. This is the scam-demic; we don't need a Bill Gates' vaccine; we need a healthy population. Take notice that Gates has never encouraged people to be healthy or emphasized that obesity and hyperglycemia play a determining role in SARS-CoV-2 infection and COVID-19 severity. Why is this? I cannot say for sure, but you should know that getting the population healthy is very bad for the business of billionaires (8).

If all Americans were healthy and fit, the novel coronavirus called SARS-CoV-2 would have passed through the population with very little ill effect. We might not have even known about it. We know this is true because it was broadly publicized that healthy people can be infected and have no symptoms *at all* or just be mildly compromised. In other words, government officials and news outlets should have sounded the alarm for Americans to get healthy because if you are healthy, you will not get COVID-19 and may even have no symptoms at all if you are infected.

Our so-called leaders could have also explained that SARS-CoV-2 infection in the obese population is very different. We could have been told that infected obese people have increased viral shedding, which means they produce more viruses and stay infected longer and are therefore highly contagious compared to healthy asymptomatic people. This is why scientists have stated that, "due to prolonged viral shedding, quarantine in obese subjects should likely be longer than normal weight individuals" (9).

With the above in mind, no matter if the lockdown was appropriate or a dramatic inappropriate overreaction, the public should have been told that during lockdown it is very important to lose weight and normalize blood glucose levels because these are the two key factors that drive COVID-19 severity. Did anyone in the government or the news media loudly sound this alarm? Of course, the answer is a very loud NO.

It is likely that many confused people will argue that the government did not know that they should have told people to lose weight, which is an absolutely incorrect notion. Consider the title of the following paper, published in 2012, which demonstrates that we have known for many years that obesity is a promoter of viral infections:

> Beck MA. Influenza and obesity: will vaccines and antivirals protect? J Infect Dis. 2012;205:172-173.
> https://www.ncbi.nlm.nih.gov/pmc/articles/PMC3244371/

Here is the conclusion to this 2012 paper: "The growing global obesity epidemic and the constant threat of an influenza pandemic necessitate that obesity should be regarded as an independent risk factor, much like advanced age, and that current vaccine strategies may need to be adjusted for this population." Fast-forward to May of 2019, when the following article was published, which was several months before the average person ever heard of coronaviruses.

> Honce R, Schultz-Cherry S. Impact of obesity on influenza A virus pathogenesis, immune response, and evolution. Front Immunol. 2019;10:1071. May 10, 2019.
> https://www.ncbi.nlm.nih.gov/pmc/articles/PMC6523028/

Pay special attention to the conclusion of this article:

> "The growing prevalence of obesity is alarming, as infection of an obese host may soon be the standard pathogenesis, instead of the well-characterized infection of a healthy-weight host. With increasing infections in the obese host, so too may the incidence of severe influenza pandemics increase as a result of increased viral shedding, and transmission and the emergence of novel viral variants. Curbing the obesity epidemic will not only improve the quality of life for those millions of people directly affected; it will also dampen the impact of obesity on infectious disease."

It should be obvious to you that scientists have known for a long time that obesity is a promoter of viral infectiousness. Did you know that obese people have increased viral shedding and viral transmission compared to non-obese people before reading this book? Most people are completely unaware of this. Instead of broadcasting this well-known fact to the general public and urging the population to lose weight and normalize blood glucose levels to get healthy, the government and its news media continuously promoted the absurd notion that infected people who are healthy and fit are the silent carriers who spread the virus. Blaming infected people who are of normal weight and healthy for asymptomatically spreading SARS-CoV is also part of the scam-demic, which will be discussed in the next section of this chapter. Hopefully Table 1 will help to paint a clearer picture about the obesity issue in relation to COVID-19.

Table 1 (As of August 4, 2020)

Country	**United States**	**Japan**	**Japan x 2.62**
Total population	330,000,000	126,000,000	330,000,000
# infected	4,830,000	41,311	108,234
Deaths	159,000	1,023	2,680
% obesity	42%	3.6%	3.6%

Notice that a whopping 42% of the US population is obese, according to the CDC (**10**), while a mere 3.6% of adult Japanese are obese. Notice that I multiplied the total Japanese population, the # infected, and deaths by a factor of 2.62 to compare the number of people that would be infected and die from COVID-19 in Japan if its population was the same as the US. I am sure that someone suffering from "mask hysteria" will claim that the Japanese are doing so much better because mask-wearing is commonplace in Japan, but that would be an exceptionally disingenuous conclusion. The difference between the two cultures is obvious. Americans are fat and sick, while the Japanese are not, which puts the American population at a far greater risk of being infected and dying from COVID-19. Clearly, COVID-19 is not a virus crisis, it is an obesity crisis. Here are the facts about the nature of viral infections in obese individuals:

1. Obese people are more prone to viral and bacterial infections (11,12)
2. Infected obese people shed more viruses (9,13)
3. Obese people create more viral mutations with increased virulence (14,15)
4. Infected obese people stay infected longer (9)
5. Infected obese people are more contagious (9)
6. Obese people have increased breathing rates and a greater exhalation volume, which leads to increased release of virus-rich aerosols without coughing or sneezing (16).
7. Vaccines are less effective in obese people compared to normal weight individuals (17,18).

If you were unaware of #s 1-7, why do you think that might be the case? In other words, why are you finding out about these facts in a self-published book as opposed to from the multibillion-dollar news media industry or the government or the health care industry? You should understand that when news outlets state that obese people are at greater risk of developing a severe case of COVID-19, it is only a small part of the story. The correct message should be that obese people are the greatest perpetuators and transmitters of the virus, and so they should be encouraged to lose body fat and normalize glucose levels. These facts lead real scientists to suggest that obese people should be quarantined longer then normal weight people (9). Why do you think that message has not been delivered to the public at large? I will give my thoughts on this topic later in this chapter.

Here is one more fact about obesity that is virtually unknown in the medical world and general population. Scientists have known since at least 1981 that people can be of normal weight and also be metabolically obese (16,19-22). These are typically non-exercisers with unhealthy muscle tissue, a non-obese fat mass that is pro-inflammatory, and high blood glucose. While viral infection studies are lacking in this population, these people are likely to have similar reactions to a viral infection as overtly obese people, as demonstrated in a recent COVID-19 study (16). This is why tracking the inflammatory markers in Chapter 4 are so important and why the DeFlame concept has such utility.

In summary, COVID-19 is a very real crisis for highly inflamed people but is mostly irrelevant for healthy people. The big scam is convincing the population that the virus is stronger than a healthy body, which it is obviously not, and that the only way to return to normal is for Bill Gates to vaccinate us all…what a crock. Maybe Donald Trump and Joe Biden should make up hats for their health policy people to wear that say *"Make America Lean and Healthy Again."* That will never happen of course because getting the population healthy is not a good business model (8).

Asymptomatic, presymptomatic, and symptomatic transmission

To be clear, the driving force behind the extensive lockdown in America and around the world was the assumption that asymptomatic people are key transmitters of the SARS-CoV-2 infection. We have been presented with the image that if we were not all locked down, asymptomatic people will infect everyone and people will die as a result. Depending on the language used to promote this notion, the image can be compelling and downright frightening, which likens SARS-CoV-2 to the fictional killer virus called Motaba in the movie *Outbreak*. In fact, the propaganda was so effective, it causes some people on social media to regularly accuse less gullible people of not caring about people if they die from COVID-19. Such hysterical accusations seem to have their basis in the belief that SARS-CoV-2 is primarily transferred by asymptomatic people.

You should understand that the degree to which asymptomatic people spread SARS-CoV-2 has yet to be determined. I know that will sound surprising to many, but it is the truth. And even if the "asymptomatic infection story" were as true as many people have been led to believe, it is important to remember that COVID-19 is not a virus crisis, it is an obesity crisis. If there was not an obesity epidemic in America, most people walking around would not know that a virus worked its way through society. There would have likely been an unfortunate uptick in deaths of sickly people in nursing homes, but that would be it, save for the occasional unfortunate outlier mortality event.

So what do you actually know about asymptomatic transmission other than the fact that news outlets have continuously beaten it into our heads that it is completely true and a terrifyingly dangerous issue? In fact, most people know very little other than what they have heard or read in the news. My perception is that asymptomatic and presymptomatic transmission has been substantially exaggerated and improperly characterized.

What does asymptomatic actually mean? It means you have absolutely no symptoms and feel great...you could even say that you never felt better. You should understand that very few middle-aged adults and older are asymptomatic – most people have aches and pains of some kind. This holds true for many lean healthy people, but it is especially the case for obese people. Even if symptoms are minor, it means that you are not asymptomatic.

Additionally, have you perhaps noticed that when "authorities" discuss asymptomatic transmission, they *never* distinguish between healthy lean people who are asymptomatic compared to overweight and obese people who claim to be asymptomatic? The fact that no authorities make this distinction automatically delegitimizes the asymptomatic transmission argument. Recall from earlier in this chapter and in Chapter 9 that the immune profile of obese people resembles that of a viral infection. So, if it is possible that asymptomatic transmission is occurring to a small degree, it is likely the unhealthy obese population is responsible for this as they are more easily infected, create more viral mutations with increased virulence, shed more viruses, are more contagious, and should be quarantined longer (9,11,12,14,15).

Here are some important facts you should understand about the nature of symptoms. First, there are two types, which are referred to as positive and negative symptoms. If you search for these on the internet, you will mostly see them in the context of schizophrenia, however they are applicable for other conditions. Some common examples of positive symptoms associated with viral infections include a sore throat, headaches, muscle aches, coughing, and difficulty breathing. No one really ever thinks about negative symptoms, as they are often so subtle. A friend of mine is particularly aware of these subtle negative symptoms. She knows she might be getting sick before she has any positive sickness symptoms at all. She learned, overtime, to recognize subtle negative symptoms, which she refers to as a *shade of a difference* compared to how she normally feels. Her typical negative symptoms include a very subtle lack of pep in her step or feeling subtly mellow and less outgoing for no reason, or just having a nebulous subtle feeling of being slightly "off." All three of these negative symptoms are just barely noticeable, which is why she describes them as feeling just a *shade of a difference* compared to normal.

These subtle negative symptoms are not terribly different from how most people feel if they do not get enough sleep, but in the case of a viral infection, they manifest when you are sleeping fine. Eventually, my friend learned to recognize her negative symptoms as a sign of potentially getting sick because she realized they manifested without a loss of sleep. When she heeds the warning of her subtle negative symptoms and rests herself, she typically does not get sick; however, if she does not rest up, she often will get sick and be in bed for a week. Most people do not recognize these symptoms or do not remember them being present after they are suffering with very positive viral infection symptoms.

There is another dilemma to overcome when dealing with the notion of asymptomatic transmission. Most obese people and normal weight people, who are metabolically obese, tend to not feel especially well on a daily basis, so they may not recognize subtle feelings of unwellness, which could otherwise alert them to the possibility that they may have a viral infection.

With the above in mind, consider the dilemma for scientists when they are trying to figure out if asymptomatic viral transmission truly occurs. Are people truly asymptomatic or do they have subtle symptoms that are ignored by patients and missed by clinicians? My impression is that doctors and patients fail to capture subtle symptoms during the initial phase of a viral infection, which means my impression is that asymptomatic SARS-CoV-2 transmission is not likely. Consider the title of the following article:

> Gao M, Yang L, Chen X, et al. A study on infectivity of asymptomatic SARS-CoV-2 carriers. Respiratory Med. 2020;169:106026. Published on May 13, 2020.
> https://www.ncbi.nlm.nih.gov/pmc/articles/PMC7219423/

The subject of this study is a 22-year old female with congenital heart disease. For 16 years, she suffered from shortness of breath, which got worse for one month prior to going to the hospital for evaluation. Her respiratory symptoms improved to preadmission status, and while at the hospital she tested positive for SARS-CoV-2, but never developed any symptoms of infection (malaise, fever, sore throat, aches and pains) or the more COVID-specific symptoms, and there was no mention of the more subtle symptoms discussed above. The researchers identified 455 people who were in contact with this asymptomatic subject and NOT a single person became infected. This very detailed contact tracing study suggests that asymptomatic people who are infected with SARS-CoV-2 probably do not transmit the infection.

With the above case in mind, consider the comments made at a World Health Organization (WHO) press conference by Dr. Maria Van Kerkhove on June 8, 2020. She explained that it is very rare for asymptomatic people to transmit the virus to others. In other words, she let the truth slip out about asymptomatic transmission (23):

> "We have a number of reports from countries who are doing very detailed contact tracing. They're following asymptomatic cases. They're following contacts. And

> they're not finding secondary transmission onward. It's very rare."

You can see that this is a very scientific statement. You can watch her in a video at CNBC's website (10) and probably on YouTube, and you will see her matter-of-fact comments about the rarity of asymptomatic transmission – she made a very simple factual statement that is consistent with the Gao study cited above. Dr. Van Kerkhove appears to be an honest doctor and so she told the truth; she is not a politician or a medical bureaucrat like Dr. Fauci. Not surprisingly, she back peddled on her statements shortly after this interview. My suspicion is that she was pressured into it and of course, Dr. Fauci jumped into the mix stating that asymptomatic viral transmission does occur (24), but where is his evidence? Sadly, Fauci lacks evidence.

Recall from Chapter 8 that I briefly described the first published report about asymptomatic transmission of SARS-CoV-2 (25). You should understand that this report was a "letter to the editor" in the *New England Journal of Medicine* (25), which is essentially meaningless when it comes to evidence in the world of science. It described a Chinese woman who travelled to Germany where she met with four business colleagues, who subsequently were infected with SARS-CoV-2 and became symptomatic. The letter stated that she did not have any symptoms while in Germany but developed them on her flight home.

This "letter to the editor" led Dr. Anthony Fauci to triumphantly claim that this study proved that asymptomatic transfer does occur, and it "lays the question to rest" (26). You have to realize that no self-respecting college student majoring in the basic sciences would make such a claim based on a "letter to the editor." So why did Dr. Fauci make such an amateurish blunder? Furthermore, why have we never seen Fauci discuss the real COVID crisis, which is rampant obesity? I suspect there are economic and social engineering reasons for this that I will discuss later in this chapter.

Real scientists finally tracked down the alleged "asymptomatic" patient from China described in the "letter to the editor" and when she was questioned, it was discovered that she did in fact have acute phase symptoms when she infected her coworkers. Her symptoms included fatigue, muscle pain, and she was taking Tylenol for her symptoms, which may have also included a low-grade fever (26). Here is the title of reference #26:

> Kupferschmidt K. Study claiming new coronavirus can be transmitted by people without symptoms was flawed. Science Magazine. February 3, 2020.
> https://www.sciencemag.org/news/2020/02/paper-non-symptomatic-patient-transmitting-coronavirus-wrong

If you go and read this article, it includes a June 2, 2020 update, which reads:

> "This story has been cited widely on social media to argue against the use of face masks and shelter-in-place policies. This is based on a misreading of the article. The fact that the New England Journal of Medicine paper had a flaw does not mean asymptomatic transmission (by people who have absolutely no symptoms) does not exist; this *is still under discussion*. But it is now well-established that people with very mild symptoms — so mild they are unlikely to recognize them as COVID-19 — can infect others and even spark large outbreaks of disease."

Because the possibility of asymptomatic transmission *is still under discussion* as of June 2020, it means that they have not demonstrated it to be a factual occurrence as I have described previously in this chapter. Also note that they emphasize the importance of mild symptoms, which I also described earlier in this chapter as a key issue to appreciate. What you should conclude at this point is that the world was locked down based on the *assumption* of asymptomatic transmission, not based on any factual evidence. Despite this fact, people believe in asymptomatic transmission. Here is an example of such a belief, which was a response to a Facebook comment I made about the problems we have with identifying if people are truly asymptomatic:

> "The hospital I used to work at just had a massive outbreak that has been definitively traced to a nurse that traveled a bit, came back, didn't quarantine, was completely asymptomatic and returned to work and unknowingly infected 36 people (physicians, other nurses, and patients on their wing) within the first couple of days back until it was discovered. Only possibility was this one nurse who had contact with all those that were infected. Asymptomatic people can definitely spread the virus."

Most people I know who go on vacation return feeling fatigued to the point they need another vacation to rest up from the vacation they just took. Some people even develop cold symptoms after a vacation. So, this quote above has to be taken with a grain of salt. My bet is that this nurse had subtle symptoms that were very mild that she probably ignored, which is very common after being on vacation. Furthermore, she probably feels terribly guilty about being the COVID transmitter and so has convinced herself that she was completely asymptomatic, which is a normal mind-protecting psychological response. You should understand that I am not writing from this point of view because I cannot accept the possibility of asymptomatic transmission – the evidence is just very weak at the moment, which I combine with my personal experience in these matters.

For about 15 years, I worked during the week and traveled 2-4 weekends per month. I would return on Sunday night and be at work on Monday morning, which I always viewed as my recovery day. I took it easy because I felt slightly less well than usual. Additionally, the way I felt on Monday precisely resembled how I would otherwise feel if I was "catching a cold." So, my position is that people are being exceptionally liberal with their definitions of asymptomatic. And this should be understood in the context that most Americans don't sleep as much or as well as they would like and most Americans also feel chronically stressed to varying degrees, so a huge number of Americans do not feel truly well as a way of life. Americans are also a heavily medicated population because we are such an unwell population…most overweight and obese people also do not feel well to varying degrees…so I would really like to know where all of these perfectly healthy asymptomatic carriers of infections are to be found.

What about presymptomatic SARS-CoV-2 transmission? These are people who are described as being infected with SARS-CoV-2 who allegedly transmit the infection before they manifest symptoms of infection, which is in contrast with asymptomatic people who are infected but never develop symptoms. You should realize from the previous discussion earlier in this chapter that symptoms of infection can be very subtle, so I have doubts about the veracity of the claim that presymptomatic people have absolutely *no symptoms* before they develop more obvious infection symptoms. I am not alone in this view. In a recent article about presymptomatic transmission, the scientists stated the following (27):

> "Identifying symptom onset relies on patient recall after confirmation of COVID-19…The potential recall bias would probably have tended toward the direction of under-ascertainment, that is, delay in recognizing first symptoms. This would cause the proportion of presymptomatic transmission to be artifactually inflated."

This means that patients, in general, are not especially reliable when it comes to precisely remembering when they started to feel sick after they are asked about it when they are in the middle of their actual sickness symptoms, which can lead to overestimating the prevalence of presymptomatic transmission. This applies to women and men, but particularly relevant for men.

You should know that men in particular are particularly unreliable when it comes rating their health status, which is very similar to rating their sickness status. Back in 2004, scientists in Sweden published an article about self-rated health and inflammation (28). In this study, 265 consecutive patients (174 women and 91 men) were asked by the authors to rate their health (excellent, very good, good, fair, or poor) and this was compared to levels of interleukin-1, a pro-inflammatory cytokine. They identified that self-rated health in women was directly correlated to IL-1 levels, while there was no correlation among male subjects. In other words, if a man cannot accurately rate his health, he is not likely to be able to accurately determine when he began to feel subtly unwell due to a viral infection, so studies published about so-called asymptomatic or presymptomatic men should be viewed as especially questionable.

You should know that there are some studies that suggest asymptomatic transmission does occur (29,30); however, these studies do not describe how they determined that the subjects were absolutely asymptomatic. The authors do not describe the criteria that was used to determine if subjects were truly asymptomatic. Did they screen for very mild symptoms? We do not know which symptoms they screened for, which is quite problematic. The June 2, 2020 clarification in *Science Magazine* made it very clear about the importance of very mild symptoms (26):

> "But it is now well-established that people with very mild symptoms—so mild they are unlikely to recognize them as COVID-19—can infect others and even spark large outbreaks of disease."

At this point, you should understand that the potential of, and degree to which, asymptomatic and presymptomatic transmission of the SARS-CoV-2 virus is occurring has NOT yet to be established by real scientists, which means that government policies have not been based on science. You should also understand that Dr. Fauci's devotion to asymptomatic transmission without evidence reflects that he has not been behaving like a scientist when it comes to COVID-19; he is clearly biased and I think there is a very obvious reason why Fauci is behaving badly. Simply stated, Dr. Fauci is a bureaucrat and lifelong bureaucrats talk out of both sides of their mouths, just like politicians. Fauci graduated from medical school, did his residency, and then immediately began working at the NIH, which means that he is a lifetime bureaucrat so he happily tows the COVID-19 party line and the related draconian lockdown that could lead to a long-lasting economic depression, perhaps worse than the one that began after the 1929 crash.

If you think the riots were/are bad after the George Floyd incident, imagine the riots that could emerge from the 40 million who lost their jobs due to months of lockdown because asymptomatic transfer is very rare, which means that a pervasive lockdown event and economic depression should have never happened in America and most other countries. No one should be surprised that Fauci, his fellow bureaucrats, and politicians will lock arms and defend their actions to avoid the wrath of multiple millions of people whose lives have been destroyed by their actions. The last thing the US government wants is to be turned on by angry political liberals and conservatives who find common ground to lock arms in outrage and then revolt against the government that put 40 million Americans out of work because of a virus that has virtually no effect on healthy and mild to moderately inflamed people.

The final scam-demic issue involves how deaths were reported. In a Whitehouse press conference on April 7, 2020, Dr. Deborah Birx made the following statement:

> "There are other countries that if you had a pre-existing condition and let's say the virus caused you to go to the ICU and then have a heart or kidney problem — some countries are recording that as a heart issue or a kidney issue and not a COVID-19 death…"The intent is...if someone dies with COVID-19, we are counting that as a COVID-19 death."

Dr. Ngozi Ezike of the Illinois Department of Health made the following statement in a press conference:

> "If someone is dying in hospice and had been given only a few weeks to live, and you were also found to have COVID, that would be counted as a COVID death...Technically if you died from a clear alternate cause, but you had COVID at the same time, it's still listed as a COVID death."
> https://www.youtube.com/watch?v=Tw9Ci2PZKZg

This means that COVID-19 deaths have been inflated to varying degrees so that we will never truly know how many people actually died from COVID-19. The perception of deaths from COVID-19 are further inflated by deceptive commentary related to the number of SARS-CoV-2 infection cases versus the number of deaths from COVID-19. In other words, the average person is led to believe that a positive test for SARS-CoV-2 means that you could easily die, which is so far from the truth it is laughable.

Imagine that all 328 million Americans were infected with SARS-CoV-2. Most people would be asymptomatic and very few would die except for the severely inflamed among us. Based on the current evidence, this is exactly what would happen. Consider the following information presented to us by Dr. John Ioannidis, which he discussed in a news outlet interview on June 27, 2020 (31): "For people younger than 45, the infection fatality rate is almost 0%. For 45 to 70, it is probably about 0.05-0.3%. For those above 70, it escalates substantially, to 1% or higher for those over 85. For frail, debilitated elderly people with multiple health problems who are infected in nursing homes, it can go up to 25% during major outbreaks in these facilities." This information is consistent with what Dr. Ioannidis wrote in a March 2020 scientific article:

Ioannidis JP. Coronavirus disease 2019: the harms of exaggerated information and non-evidence-based measures. Eur J Clin Invest. 2020;50:e13222
https://onlinelibrary.wiley.com/doi/full/10.1111/eci.13222

Clearly, the obvious fact is that most people would get through a SARS-CoV-2 infection without ill-effect. Unfortunately, this truth is not reported. Instead the misleading reporting causes our minds to conflate the number of cases with the number of poor outcomes, which falsely inflates the number of deaths in people's minds to create the illusion that SARS-CoV-2 is lethal across the board.

By inflating the numbers in this fashion described above, in addition to the subliminal promotion that SARS-CoV-2 is as bad as Motaba from the movie *Outbreak*, the government has the fuel it needs to engage in draconian lockdown measures. I do not understand why lockdown is so important to them and could only speculate as to why. But I can tell you something very interesting that definitely happened between January and June of 2020, and it involves the troubled US and world economy.

An economic theory about lockdown and social unrest

In November of 2008, Rahm Emanuel, who was to be President Obama's chief of staff stated, "you never want a serious crisis to go to waste, and what I mean by that is that it is an opportunity to do things you think you could not do before." You should understand that this is not a democrat-specific ideology. It is a political ideology that republicans also engage in, as well as monarchs and oligarchs in other countries.

It should not be a surprise to anyone that the world economy has struggled for years, which became blatantly obvious during the 2008 financial crisis, to which Emanuel's comment was referring. The movie called *The Big Short* did an excellent job of portraying what happened in the housing market that caused the so-called Great Recession, which involved the creation of toxic financial instruments called mortgage-backed securities that spun out of control.

Fast forward to January 2020 at the World Economic Forum in Davos, Switzerland. An attendee named Scott Minerd was interviewed, who is the Chief Investment Officer at Guggenheim which manages over $260 billion in assets, so this guy is clearly no lightweight. Minerd explained that we live in a Ponzi-like economy, which has been going on in an accelerated fashion since about 1980, which also means that it existed before 1980.

At the time of the Minerd interview in January of 2020, COVID-19 was not yet a big issue and there were no protests and rioting going on. Then, between January and June of 2020 during the COVID crisis, protests, and riots, the Federal Reserve bank took on over $3 trillion in assets (32), which is a euphemistic way of saying it took on toxic debt or toxic assets, much of which are mortgage-backed securities from at risk banks. In other words, this was the biggest bank bailout in the history of mankind, and mostly no one knows about it.

You should understand that the Federal Reserve essentially runs our American Ponzi economy and has great influence around the world because the US dollar has been the world's reserve currency since World War II ended. Read up on the Bretton Woods Conference if you would like more details. Since the Federal Reserve is in charge of our Ponzi economy, you should not be surprised if they participate or weigh in on the lockdown. Not surprisingly, on August 2, 2020, Reuters published an article entitled:

> Fed's Kashkari suggests 4-6 week shutdown; says U.S. Congress can spend big on coronavirus relief (33)

Neel Kashkari is the President of the Minneapolis Federal Reserve Bank and he stated that, "the U.S. economy could benefit if the nation were to 'lock down really hard' for four to six weeks...Congress can well afford large sums for coronavirus relief efforts." So, it should be obvious who is driving our current economic and social reality into the abyss...bankers, bureaucrats, incompetent politicians, and science bureaucrats. Here is a bit more information about the Federal Reserve.

The way the Federal Reserve buys debt and other "assets" is to literally type "dollars" into their computers and use it to buy mortgage-backed securities, bonds, etc. This is why this process is criticized as "printing money out of thin air." Imagine typing into existence $3 trillion dollars in just 6 months and using it to "buy" up assets…amazing. This took the Federal Reserve's balance sheet from about $4 trillion to $7 trillion worth of assets bought with "money" it created out of thin air. The Federal Reserve is also typing up currency in the billions to buy corporate bonds to ensure that huge corporations do not fail, which keeps the stock market from crashing to create the illusion of prosperity. Did you know about these activities?

Most people do not know what the Federal Reserve is doing because we have been distracted by COVID-19, heightened social unrest, and the Jeffrey Epstein underaged sex trafficking scandal. Most people also do not know that the shady activity of bankers led to them being broadly referred to as "banksters" in the early 1900s. And finally, very few people know that Thomas Jefferson warned us about private central banks, explaining that private banking institutions are more detrimental to freedom and liberty than standing foreign armies.

The Fed, as the Federal Reserve is called, has previously typed $3 trillion dollars into existence; it just did it more slowly over time. This occurred between 2008 and 2014 when they "typed" up $3 trillion dollars to deal with the housing crisis fallout, which increased the Fed's asset accumulation from $1 trillion to $4 trillion. It is important to understand that this typing/buying activity took place in response to the bursting of the housing bubble in 2008.

The question I would like answered is: "What financial crisis happened during 2019 that caused the Fed to type up $3 trillion in just 6 months?" We are not likely to find out the answer to this question, but I think Scott Minerd encapsulated it well. Because we live in a Ponzi-like economy, such actions are required from time to time to keep the Ponzi scheme going, and a pandemic scare and social unrest can be used as a good cover to bail out the so-called "too big to fail banks."

For those who do not know, the Federal Reserve is a private banking institution from which the US government borrows money at interest, which is why the US national debt grows every year. I should qualify the word "borrow" because it does not mean what you think. For example, if I were to borrow $200 from you, the only way that would work is if you had $200 that you could lend me. You could not type $200 onto a piece of paper and give it to me. Similarly, you could not transfer $200 to my bank account unless you had $200 in your account. This is not how the US government "borrows" money from the Federal Reserve.

When the US government needs currency to operate beyond what taxes bring in, the Fed is contacted, which then creates the needed currency units by typing them into a computer. These currency unit dollars are then loaned to the US government with interest on currency that did not exist in the first place. This is another example of why the term "printing money out of thin air" is used when describing the relationship between the US government and the Federal Reserve. If this seems shocking, you should know that the same process is involved when the average person takes out a "loan" from a commercial bank to buy a house or other big-ticket item.

Before most of you bought your house, the "dollars" to buy the house did not exist. The "dollars" were created "out of thin air" by the bank to create your mortgage by typing US currency units called dollars into a computer, and now you owe interest on currency/money that did not otherwise exist before you signed on the dotted line for the mortgage.

Do you have a student loan? If you do, you should know that you are the one who created the currency to pay for college when you signed the student loan document. In other words, the money to pay for your college tuition did not exist until you signed it into existence. Almost all so-called "loans" from banks work like this. They are not really loans. If you did not know this, it should cause you to ask what else do you not know?

This same process is at work when you use your credit card. Your credit limit really refers to the amount of currency you are allowed to create out of thin air when you swipe your card, which you owe back with interest. What an amazing business model for the owners of the banks.

The above examples should help to explain why governments and individuals are awash in debt. "Money" is created out of thin air at interest, so there is more debt in existence than actual currency. There is obviously a limit to which you and I can do this, but the US government does this with the Federal Reserve in an unlimited-like fashion, which is why they together are running a massive Ponzi scheme. The US government never has enough currency units (dollars/money) it needs to run all its programs and departments because it is technically broke. To not default and to keep all of its programs and departments going, the US government keeps borrowing currency, created out of thin air at interest by the Fed. If you do an internet search for "US treasury national debt by year" this is the first hit you will get:

www.treasurydirect.gov › ... › Public Debt Reports ▾

Government - Historical Debt Outstanding – Annual

Feb 4, 2020 - **TreasuryDirect** Logo. You are in ... Historical **Debt** Outstanding – Annual. 2000 - 2019 · 1950 - 1999 ... The **History of the Debt**. Our Heritage ...

2000 - 2019 · 1790 - 1849 · Annual 1950 - 1999 · 1850 - 1899

It is important to understand that treasurydirect.gov is an official US government website that keeps a historical record of the US government debt. Wars typically involve massive debt expansion, which is obvious during the World War II era. Otherwise, US government debt increased gradually, which means it was a slow-growing Ponzi-economy; that is until 1981 when Ronald Reagan took office. Table 1 outlines US monetary inflation (debt expansion) from 1950 to 2020.

Table 1 - US debt expansion from 1981 to 2020

Presidential era	US National Debt Expansion
Years 1950-1977	$255 billion to $650 billion
Carter (1977-1980)	$650 billion to $1 trillion
Reagan (1981-1988)	$1 to $3 trillion
Bush (1989-1991)	$3 to $4 trillion
Clinton (1992-2000)	$4 to $5.5 trillion
Bush (2001-2008)	$5.5 to $10 trillion
Obama (2009-2016)	$10 to $20 trillion
Trump (2017-June 2020)	$20 to $26 trillion

I pulled the information in Table 1 from the US government's treasurydirect website mentioned above. You should know that I rounded the numbers for easier reading. You should also understand, and never forget, that the presidents listed in Table 1 are figureheads; they do not control monetary policy. So, blaming a president for our economic woes is not accurate. No matter who was president from 1950 to 2020, we would have likely had the same government currency creation and debt expansion. In other words, a president in office merely observes the currency expansion and national debt growth that would have happened whether or not he was in office.

There are a few notable points to mention about Table 1, which will be stressful to you if you are a republican/democrat and believe what republicans/democrats in office tell you. What I am about to describe is based on the US government's actual debt numbers listed in Table 1.

First, consider that Ronald Reagan is still loved today by republicans. Reagan presented himself like a small government guy and a fiscal conservative and his fans still believe this; however, Table 1 demonstrates the opposite to be the case. Save for FDR's debt expansion, no president other than Ronald Reagan oversaw a tripling of the US national debt, which means that Reagan was not fiscally conservative or a promoter of a smaller government.

Second, consider also that Bill Clinton is still loved today by democrats. Clinton claimed that he left office with a surplus; however, Table 2 demonstrates that there was no surplus. In fact, an additional $1.5 trillion was added to the national debt during the Clinton era. The lie that Bill Clinton balanced the budget and left a multibillion-dollar surplus is still believed by democrats to this day.

Understand that I chose to highlight the Reagan and Clinton examples to illustrate two obvious misconceptions that are harbored by many. If you did not know these economic details, an appropriate follow-up thought should be..."what else am I unaware of" or "what else have I been led to believe that is erroneous" or "how else have I been lied to." In the context of COVID-19, it is likely that you did not know a lot about what was previously discussed in this book, so my thinking that COVID-19 and social unrest is being used as cover to rejigger the financial system should not be viewed as a stretch.

Fast forward from the Reagan and Clinton eras to 2020 where we now have a $26 trillion national debt and massive toxic debt accumulation by the Federal Reserve. This unpayable Ponzi economy debt accumulation has been fostered for decades by corrupt politicians and a corrupt banking system. This fact is ignored by our corrupt media industrial complex and instead we are told that economy suffers due to various unforeseen crises that emerge like black swans, the most recent being COVID-19 and social unrest.

The "powers that shouldn't be" are well aware of the problem with the US and world economy. They all know that what Scott Minerd said is true, which is why various economic "leaders" have been talking about a monetary reset in recent years to address the various toxic imbalances in our current system. Most recently this occurred in

2020 at the World Economic Forum in Davos, Switzerland. Indeed, Kristalina Georgieva, Managing Director at the International Monetary Fund, gave a presentation entitled *The Great Reset* (34).

Consider how bizarre this situation is. Over 40 million Americans lost their jobs because the economy was locked down for the COVID-19 crisis, which was only a crisis for heavily inflamed young and middle-aged people and the unwell elderly. And which people lost their jobs during this "crisis?" People who were deemed to be "non-essential" by politicians, while these same politicians and their banker and international corporation buddies, have benefited massively from the Ponzi economy that they have perpetuated…talk about elitism. These same people even increased their wealth during the lockdown to the tune of $434 billion between March and May of 2020 (35), while the average person continues to struggle with their mortgage or rent and other bills, or worse went bankrupt.

These same elitists who are responsible for, and benefited from, our Ponzi economy are the ones now calling it out as a problem as if they had nothing to do with it. And worse, the reset they are planning for will benefit themselves and not the average person who lost their job because of our Ponzi economy. Unfortunately, it seems to me that most Americans are unaware of this, and I think it is because the average person lives in a chronic state of fear and worry as each crisis consistently rolls through society every 2-4 years, which completely captures the attention of the average person. The average person is also plagued by the manufactured left-right political ideologies that magnify the fear and worry and attention.

At the present time, the average person is emerging from being locked down and trying to figure out how to live in this so-called "new corona normal," while many simultaneously still worry about dying from COVID-19 that is propagandized to be as deadly as Motaba from *Outbreak*, during which we are coincidently treated to watching brutal riots on many news channels while we sit around overeating refined sugar, flour, and oils that will make us sicker and more dependent on medications. These are very stressful issues for the body and mind to deal with, which is why I thought back in early 2020 that the second phase of the COVID-19 lockdown will be worse than the first.

In short, you should consider the very real possibility that the current crises are being created, and/or promoted, and/or exaggerated by those who control our Ponzi economy and wish to reset it in their best interest and are actually calling it *The Great Reset*. If you have never considered this as a possibility, the first reaction is to reject it, which is fine. No matter if you reject this information or not, one fact is abundantly clear; the average common person in US and most other nations is in for several years of economic uncertainty.

These same common people are awash in debt; they are slaves to their debt, which is why the term debt slavery emerged. The vast majority of Americans fall into this category to varying degrees, and these same people are justifiably angry about the massive banker bailouts that went on in 2008 and now in 2020. But there is a reason for such bailouts.

You may or may not recall the terms "too big to fail" and "too big to jail" when referring to investment banks. This was language that was used after the 2008 investment banking crisis, wherein a huge investment bank called Lehman Brothers failed due to their poor investment making. Thereafter, the US government, via the Federal Reserve, created the TARP bailout program to save other investment banks from going under. People do not realize that this has to happen in a Ponzi economy, lest the entire economic and financial system would fail. In short, the credit/debt system has to constantly expand, or the system will fail, which is why it is that we have a Ponzi economy.

Ponzi systems cannot last forever, which is why we do need an economic reset; however, this reset should not be a mirror image of the current system, which financially enslaves those in the middle class who have access to credit and keeps impoverished those in the lower income class who do not have access to credit and often rely on payday-type loans to stay afloat.

To you give you an idea of a currency system that was not created out of thin air and "loaned" to governments by private central banks with interest, we can look to historical England, which used Tally Sticks as an interest-free currency for about 700 years, which were the most prosperous years in England's history that virtually no one knows about. At their peak, Tally Sticks were used for about 95% of all financial transactions. You should not be surprised that you likely have never heard of Tally Sticks, as such information would lead the US population to direct their focus on the real economic problem that plagues America and those who are the current perpetuators of it. This 9-minute video by Bill Still explains the Tally Stick story:

https://www.youtube.com/watch?v=CQVAabQ0JcM

You should also realize that it is NOT the so-called 1% of income earners who are responsible for our current economic situation. To be in the top 1% you need to make $450,000 per year, which is obviously a lot of money. These people can clearly live very well, but they are not responsible for driving our Ponzi economy. Rather, they have managed to successfully navigate our Ponzi economy. However, these are not people who are driving around town or flying around the country oppressing the less affluent and the poor. The link below will take you to CNN Money, where you can look at where you fall in the income rankings.

https://money.cnn.com/calculator/pf/income-rank/index.html

Whoever started the anti-1% movement either is ignorant or is part of the .01% income bracket or greater and looking to avoid public scrutiny. Either way, the anti-1% movement does not remotely get at dealing with our Ponzi economic system that truly serves only a select group of superrich people who benefit greatly, while people in the middle and lower-income brackets suffer as our corrupt economic system cycles between currency inflation and deflation.

Herd immunity and the vaccine business model

In the July 7, 2020 issue of *The Wall Street Journal,* we are told that the US government gave a total of $2 billion to two drug manufacturers (Novavax and Regeneron) to develop a COVID-19 vaccine (36). After reading this book, it should be obvious that COVID-19 is a health crisis and NOT a virus crisis or an "in need of a vaccine crisis." If Americans were healthy, SARS-CoV-2 would have spread through society in a mostly unnoticed fashion, save for the unhealthy elderly population. In such a scenario, quarantine measures should have only applied to the unhealthy elderly at risk.

As states in America begin to reopen, we are likely to be inundated with propaganda about the need to create herd immunity against COVID-19. You should understand that the call for herd immunity is a call for widespread vaccination. Most people do not realize that herd immunity is a vaccine concept. An article in WebMD explains that when lots of people in an area are vaccinated, fewer people get sick, which means there are fewer germs to spread around from person to person – this is called herd immunity (37).

If SARS-CoV-2 caused severe COVID-19 in every infected person, then it would be reasonable to create a vaccine, but we know that most people are mildly affected by the infection or have no idea they are infected. So why are they pushing the herd immunity/vaccine issue? We have to remember that getting people healthy is bad for the business of billionaires (8), and it is also bad for our dysfunctional economy.

Imagine if the medical industrial complex and the government loudly sounded the alarm to Americans that we all need to get lean and healthy to the point where our blood glucose levels were below 90 mg/dL and there was no more obesity. Even further, how would you feel if the government mandated that we achieve a normal weight and normal glucose levels? The fact that they can mandate mask-wearing, social distancing, beach closures, and bankrupt small businesses, they could certainly mandate normal blood glucose and body weight for the general welfare of the people. Most people would lose their minds if there was a normal weight/glucose mandate, but many happily accept the mask mandate.

If we all achieved a normal body weight and glucose levels below 90 mg/dL, then virtually no one would suffer from COVID-19 and the vaccine issue would be irrelevant. But there is a reason why the government would never mandate getting healthy; because it would mean that most people would have to stop buying soda, desserts, candy, and refined flour products like white bread. This change in buying habits would partially or substantially collapse the US economy, as most Americans get 60% of their calories from refined sugar, flour, and oils. Getting Americans healthy would also mean that Novavax and Regeneron would not get their created out-of-thin-air $2 billion to perpetuate the Ponzi economy.

With the above information in mind, it should be obvious why they are going to use fear and shaming techniques to push the herd immunity/vaccine issue; it's all about keeping the Ponzi going. Voices that object to being vaccinated will be met with typical criticisms – such people will be criticized for being anti-science, anti-medicine, anti-government conspiracy theorists, and worse, they will be criticized for being hateful people who do not care about their fellow humans. All of this is nonsense of course, but it will likely happen nonetheless and be promoted by the government and its media, AND by many in the confused public who have been tricked into believing that COVID-19 is a virus crisis, when it is actually a health/obesity crisis.

What you can do

The average person, which is most of us, will not be involved in whatever reset may be coming, so what should you do? We can all certainly learn more about our controlling economic and political systems, so as to stop falling for the Left-Right political propaganda, which hurts the vast majority of people who incorrectly think that the next president or member of congress will fix the system.

Protests and anger should be directed toward the elitists who control and perpetuate our corrupt systems, rather than fellow citizens, most of whom are just trying to make ends meet and keep their lives from falling apart. But more important is to make yourself and loved ones as mentally and physically resilient as possible, which involves improving body health.

The last thing one needs during a protracted period of economic turmoil is a chronically inflamed body, which will only add to the one's personal economic stress. This is why we all need to DeFlame ourselves to the best of our ability, which involves DeFlaming the diet, taking supplements that reduce inflammation, staying active, getting adequate sleep, and avoiding unnecessary stressors.

Another consideration is to grow food on your property. No matter the climate, food can be grown, so figure out what grows best in your area and start planting your yard. I can say for sure that potatoes of all varieties provide the best bang for your buck, so that is a place to start. A couple of years ago in my yard, there was only grass and weeds that grew into trees. I cleared the land and planted only food trees and pollinator plants/trees. You can do the same, no matter the size of your property.

Mass mask hysteria

You may have noticed the obvious fact that I have written absolutely nothing about masks, hand washing, and social distancing. My reason for writing about mask-wearing in the final paragraphs of the final chapter of this book is because it should be obvious now that healthy people really do not need to worry much even if they do get infected because it is only the exceptionally inflamed middle-aged population or the frail and sick older population that suffer from complications and death. Furthermore, my mother taught me about staying away from sick people (social distancing - although we did not call it that) and washing my hands when I was 5 years old or younger. So these two suggestions are exceptionally elementary. I learned about them when I was in kindergarten or earlier, which means they are literally "elementary" recommendations.

Mask wearing is also rather elementary, but relatively new for Americans, so I suppose the novelty has inflated its alleged importance and led to confusion in the minds of the poorly informed pro- and anti-maskers. I have tested this out in Facebook when people post anti- or pro-mask comments. Without taking a pro- or anti-mask position, I posted the following quote from a commentary written by an infectious disease expert at Harvard with over 200 published papers.

> "We know that wearing a mask outside health care facilities offers little, if any, protection from infection. Public health authorities define a significant exposure to COVID-19 as face-to-face contact within 6 feet with **symptomatic COVID-19** that is sustained for at least a few minutes (and some say more than 10 minutes or even 30 minutes). The chance of catching COVID-19 from a passing interaction in a public space is therefore minimal. In many cases, the desire for widespread masking is a reflexive reaction to anxiety over the pandemic." (38)

I thought such a statement would calm the minds of pro- and anti-maskers alike because it provides an orientation for mask-wearing in the context of becoming infected. However, to my surprise, when I posted this on a pro-masker's thread, I was accused of being an anti-masker. Similarly, when I posted this on an anti-masker's thread, I was accused of being a pro-masker. This should help you to understand that few people understand the mask-wearing evidence. In other words, neither the pro- or anti-maskers have a metric for mask-wearing; both positions are based on emotion.

While I was writing this final chapter, a friend of mine who lives in south Florida told me that he was walking on the beach down by the ocean. He was the only person on the beach at the time - it was completely vacant except for him - however, that did not stop a beach patrolman from driving over on his 4-wheeler to tell my friend he had to be wearing a mask if he wanted to walk on the absolutely vacant beach. Similarly, I regularly see people driving in their cars by themselves while wearing masks. Do they actually think that SARS-CoV-2 is waiting for them at stop signs or somehow living in their cars? Who got into their heads to make them believe that they should wear a mask in their cars when they are alone? This represents mask hysteria.

Regarding mask-wearing, you should know that according to the CDC, SARS-CoV-2 is spread largely through respiratory droplets when an infected person coughs or sneezes (39). There is an exception to this rule and it involves the obese population. Obese people exhale a greater volume air, which leads to increased aerosol production and a greater chance to infect others around them without coughing or sneezing (16). This suggests that the obese population should be educated very carefully about the nature of mild symptoms associated with COVID-19.

It is important to understand that asymptomatic people do not have acute phase symptoms and they do not cough or sneeze because, if they did, they would clearly be symptomatic. Recall from earlier in this chapter that 455 contacts did not become infected when they were around the asymptomatic 22-year old with congenital heart disease who was infected with SARS-CoV-2. The likely reason for this is that she was not coughing and sneezing on people. Perhaps this is the reason why a June 5, 2020 report from the World Health Organization (WHO) stated (40):

> "At present, there is no direct evidence (from studies on COVID-19 and in healthy people in the community) on the effectiveness of universal masking of healthy people in the community to prevent infection with respiratory viruses, including COVID-19."

Similarly, infectious disease specialists from Down Under stated (41):

> "In Australia and New Zealand currently, the questionable benefits arguably do not justify health-care staff wearing surgical masks when treating low-risk patients and may impede the normal caring relationship between patients, parents, and staff. We counsel against such practice, at least at present."

Finally, another study that involved scientists from Harvard, the University of Maryland, and the University of Hong Kong concluded that (42), "our results indicate that surgical face masks could prevent transmission of human coronaviruses and influenza viruses from **symptomatic** individuals." They also examined virus shedding in exhaled breath from infected people with symptoms. Rhinovirus was detected in aerosols in 19 of 34 subjects, compared to 4 of 10 for coronavirus (not SARS-CoV-2) and 8 of 23 for influenza (43). We can conclude two positive findings from this study. First, masks do appear to prevent transmission from symptomatic people, and second, and even better, 56% or less patients with viral infections shed the virus in exhaled breath.

I think the sticking point for the pro-maskers is that they strongly believe that asymptomatic people are the primary drivers of the so-called pandemic for two main reasons. First, they do not understand the difference between being truly asymptomatic and having very subtle infection symptoms. Second, the asymptomatic transmission propaganda is presented 24/7 on the news and most people are unaware of Dr. Fauci's substantial error about the validity of asymptomatic transmission. Recall from earlier in this chapter that asymptomatic transmission was allegedly fully established by a "Letter to the Editor" in the *New England Journal of Medicine* (25), which Fauci applauded (26):

> "There's no doubt after reading [the *NEJM*] paper that asymptomatic transmission is occurring," Anthony Fauci,

> director of the U.S. National Institute of Allergy and Infectious Diseases, told journalists. "This study lays the question to rest."

First, the "letter" was not a paper based on a detailed study – shame on Fauci. Second, the authors of the letter failed to contact the alleged asymptomatic patient to determine if she actually had any symptoms of infection. When the alleged "asymptomatic" patient was questioned, it was discovered that she did have infection symptoms when she infected her coworkers. She felt tired, suffered from muscle pain, might have had a fever, and was taking Tylenol (26). In other words, the alleged asymptomatic patient was actually symptomatic when she transferred the infection. Dr Fauci has clearly failed us all.

Because people are so emotional about mask wearing, I want to make it clear that I am not taking an anti- or pro-mask position. My position could best be described as being "when-mask" or "who-mask." In other words, we need objective information about SARS-CoV-2 transmission so that proper mask-wearing criteria can be developed. Slogans to promote mask-wearing are not helpful in this regard and neither are shaming tactics to promote compliance. So, in conclusion, what does the science tell us about SARS-CoV-2 and COVID-19? Here are some considerations.

1. We know that COVID-19 is a health/obesity crisis. Obese people are more easily infected, shed more viruses, more readily mutate viruses, stay infected longer, and are more contagious.
2. Normal weight individuals can be metabolically obese. In theory, these people are as infectious as obese individuals.
3. We do not know for sure if there is asymptomatic transmission of SARS-CoV-2, and if there is such a thing, we do not know how much it occurs. It appears that for an infected person to transmit the infection, they must at least have subtle or very mild symptoms.

4. People should be educated about the subtle and very mild symptoms of a viral infection, which can lead to better self-patrolling, self-care, and proper mask-wearing.
5. Perhaps half of symptomatic virus-infected people do not release viruses in exhaled droplets or aerosols, which means we should not necessarily freak out if we only transiently have contact with an infected person.
6. Remember, that "public health authorities define a significant exposure to COVID-19 as face-to-face contact within 6 feet with **symptomatic COVID-19** that is sustained for at least a few minutes (and some say more than 10 minutes or even 30 minutes). The chance of catching COVID-19 from a passing interaction in a public space is therefore minimal" (20).
7. Symptomatic people should wear masks when around non-infected people.
8. Symptomatic people should stay home and avoid contact with others.
9. Non-infected people should wear masks if they come in contact with symptomatic infected people who should be sheltering at home or in a medical facility if need be.
10. There is no reason to wear masks when outdoors or in your car or walking through stores unless they are crowded, so in the case of stores, have one with you.
11. People who feel anxious about not wearing masks should wear masks if they want AND they should not deliver negative attitudes towards those who choose not to.
12. Avoid people who feel sick because they may be manifesting COVID-19 symptoms without knowing it.
13. If you feel even minimally sick, you should avoid people, self-quarantine, wear a mask if you go out around people, and get tested if you can.
14. Sneezing and coughing are the primary mechanisms by which viruses are spread, so avoid people who are sneezing and coughing. If you are sneezing and coughing, you should avoid people and stay at home, and see your medical doctor if

symptoms become more severe. If you have to go out in public, where a mask and stay away from other people.

15. Obese people exhale a greater volume air, which leads to increased aerosol production and a greater chance to infect others around them without coughing or sneezing, which suggests that mask wearing should be focused on the obese population.
16. Most obese people, and normal weight people who are metabolically obese, tend to not feel especially well on a daily basis, so they may not recognize subtle feelings of unwellness, which could otherwise alert them to the possibility that they may have a viral infection.
17. As we enter the fall/winter of 2020/2021 many obese people will have added more weight during the lockdown, referred to as the Quarantine 15, which can be potentially catastrophic because this is when the flu virus will join the Coronavirus.

If local and federal governments understood 1-17, they could have instituted a measured lockdown to help protect those at greatest risk and delivered appropriate mask-wearing recommendations to the rest of us, while simultaneously encouraging the overweight and obese population to lose body fat and get healthy. Instead, the broad draconian lockdown measures directed inappropriately at healthy people have essentially wrecked the middle class and shut down multiple small businesses, and the mask hysteria that now exists has only served to increase the mental/emotional stress within the population. Meanwhile the obese population has been placed at greater risk as Coronavirus season will soon merge with the flu season.

Hysterical promoters of universal mask-wearing do not, unfortunately, take the above information into consideration and they are also obviously unaware of the information in the first 13 chapters of this book. These people have been tricked into visualizing that we are walking around breathing deadly viruses all over each other, which is not the case at all. These are the confused mask-wearers you may have watched on the news picketing the government for greater second-phase lockdown measures for the majority of the population who will never be compromised by COVID-19. Without knowing it, these picketers for lockdown are demanding that lower income Americans be further financially compromised (43). Indeed, millions will remain out of work and millions will not be able to keep up with their mortgage payments (44). Never in my life did I expect to see people picketing for the financial demise of their fellow citizens and country at large.

It should be clear that phrases such as "staying home for the greater good" and "wear your mask to be courteous to others" are really meaningless and counterproductive when you realize that SARS-CoV-2 should have passed through the world with only a minor blip on the disease radar, which means that tens of millions of livelihoods would not have been put at risk for financial devastation. Additionally, polls suggest that up to 50% of people in lockdown have gotten fatter, which is why the term "quarantine 15" emerged (45). In short, the lockdown and fear mongering has devasted the financial lives of many people, while simultaneously causing millions to emerge from lockdown more inflamed and at a greater risk for dying from COVID-19 and the flu.

COVID-19 is a health/obesity crisis and NOT a virus crisis. If you are unhealthy, now is the time to get healthy. And if you are healthy, you should stay healthy and assist others to do the same.

References

1. https://www.newsweek.com/dr-fauci-backed-controversial-wuhan-lab-millions-us-dollars-risky-coronavirus-research-1500741
2. Wells WA. When is a virus and exosome? J Cell Biol. 2003;162:960.
3. Crenshaw BJ, Gu L, Sims B, Matthews QL. Exosome biogenesis and biological function in response to viral infections. The Open Virology J. 2018;12:134-48.
4. Hoen EN, Cremer T, Gallo RC, Margolis LB. Extracellular vesicles and viruses: are they close relatives. PNAS. 2016;113:9155-61.
5. https://www.yahoo.com/news/thought-coronavirus-fake-crisis-then-163213420.html
6. https://www.healio.com/news/endocrinology/20200520/obesity-triples-odds-of-more-severe-symptoms-with-covid19

7. Brufsky A. Hyperglycemia, hydroxychloroquine, and the COVID-19 pandemic. J Med Virol. 2020;92:770-75.
8. https://www.cnbc.com/2018/04/11/goldman-asks-is-curing-patients-a-sustainable-business-model.html
9. Luzi L, Radaelli MG. Influenza and obesity: its odd relationship and the lessons for COVID-19 pandemic. Acta Diabetologica. 2020;57:759-64.
10. CDC. Adult obesity facts. Obesity is a common, serious, and costly disease. https://www.cdc.gov/obesity/data/adult.html
11. Ghilotti F, Bellocco R, Ye W, et al. Obesity and risk of infections: results from men and women is the Swedish National March cohort. Inter J Epidemiol. 2019;48:1783-94.
12. Dhurandhar NV, Bailey D, Thomas D. Interaction of obesity and infections. Obesity Rev. 2015;16:1017-29.
13. Maier HE, Lopez R, Sanchez N, et al. Obesity increases the duration of influenza A virus shedding in adults. J Infectious Dis. 2018;218:1378-82.
14. Honce R, Schultz-Cherry S. Impact of obesity on influenza A virus pathogenesis, immune response, and evolution. Front Immunol. 2019;10:1071.
15. Honce R, Karlsson EA, Wohlegmuth N, et al. Obesity-related microenvironment promotes emergence of virulent influenza virus strains. 2020;11(2):e03341-19.
16. De Lorenzo A, Tarsitano MG, Falcone C, et al. Fat mass affects nutritional status of ICU COVID-19 patients. J Trans Med. 2020;18:299
17. Beck MA. Influenza and obesity: will vaccines and antivirals protect? J Infect Dis. 2012;205:172-173.
18. Kim YH, Kim JK, Kim DJ, et al. Diet-induced obesity dramatically reduces the efficacy of a 2009 pandemic H1N1 vaccine in a mouse model. 2012;205:244-51.
19. Ruderman NB, Schneider SC, Berchtold P. The "metabolically obese," normal-weight concept. Am J Clin Nutr. 1981;34:1617-21.
20. Ruderman N, Chisholm D, Pi-Sunyer X, Schneider S. The metabolically obese, normal-weight individual revisited. Diabetes. 1998;47:699-713.
21. St-Onge MP, Janssen K, Heymsfield S. Metabolic syndrome in normal-weight Americans. Diabetes Care. 2004;27:2222-28.
22. Teixeira TF, Alves RD, Moreira AP, Peluzio M. Main characteristics of metabolically obese normal weight and metabolically healthy obese phenotypes. Nutr Rev. 2015;73:175-90.
23. Dr. Maria Van Kerkhove interview. https://www.cnbc.com/2020/06/08/asymptomatic-coronavirus-patients-arent-spreading-new-infections-who-says.html
24. Fauci says asymptomatic coronavirus transmission is possible following WHO confusion. https://www.foxnews.com/health/fauci-says-asymptomatic-coronavirus-transmission-is-possible-following-who-statement-that-was-not-correct
25. Rothe C, Schunk M, Sothmann P, et al. Transmission of 2019-nCoV infection from an asymptomatic contact in Germany. N Eng J Med. 2020;382:970-71.
26. Kupferschmidt K. Study claiming new coronavirus can be transmitted by people without symptoms was flawed. Science Magazine. February 3, 2020.

https://www.sciencemag.org/news/2020/02/paper-non-symptomatic-patient-transmitting-coronavirus-wrong
27. He X, Lau EH, Wu P, et al. Temporal dynamics in viral shedding and transmissibility of COVID-19. Nature Med. 2020;26:672-75.
28. Lekander M, Leofsson S, Neve IM, et al. Self-rated health is related to levels of circulating cytokines. Psychosomatic Med. 2004;66:559-63.
29. Huang L, Zhang X, Zhang X, et al. Rapid asymptomatic transmission of COVID-19 during the incubation period demonstrating strong infectivity in a cluster of youngsters aged 16-23 years outside Wuhan and characteristics of young patients with COVID-19: a prospective contact-tracing study. J Infection. 2020;80:e1-e13.
30. Szablewski CM, Chang KT, Brown MM, et al. SARS-CoV-2 transmission and infection among attendees of an overnight camp—Georgia, June 2020. MMWR. 2020;69:1023-25.
31. Claus P. Up to 300 million people may be infected by COVID-19 Stanford guru John Ioannidis says. Greek Reporter. June 27, 2020. https://usa.greekreporter.com/2020/06/27/up-to-300-million-people-may-be-infected-by-covid-19-stanford-guru-john-ioannidis-says/
32. Federal Reserve printing/typing up currency: https://www.federalreserve.gov/monetarypolicy/bst_recenttrends.htm
33. Reuters. Fed's Kashkari suggests 4-6 shutdown; says U.S. Congress can spend big on coronavirus relief. https://www.reuters.com/article/us-health-coronavirus-fed/feds-kashkari-suggests-4-6-week-shutdown-says-us- congress-can-spend-big-on-coronavirus-relief-idUSKBN24Y0IM
34. World Economic Forum. The great reset: https://www.imf.org/en/News/Articles/2020/06/03/sp060320-remarks-to-world-economic-forum-the-great-reset
35. Frank R. American billionaires got $434 billion richer during the pandemic. CNBC. May 21, 2020. https://www.cnbc.com/2020/05/21/american-billionaires-got-434-billion-richer-during-the-pandemic.html
36. Loftus P, Walker J. US commits $2 billion for COVID-19 vaccine, drug supplies. The Wall Street Journal. July 7, 2020. https://www.wsj.com/articles/u-s-commits-2-billion-for-covid-19-vaccine-drug-supplies-11594132175
37. Watson S. What's herd immunity and how does it protect us? WebMD. Dec 3, 2018. https://www.webmd.com/vaccines/news/20181130/what-herd-immunity-and-how-does-it-protect-us
38. Klompas M, Morris CA, Sinclair J, et al. Universal masking in hospitals in the Covid-19 eral. N Eng J Med. 2020;382:e63.
39. Hendrix MJ, Walde C, Findley K, Trotman R. Absence of apparent transmission of SARS-CoV-2 from two stylists after exposure at a hair salon with a universal face covering policy—Springfield, Missouri, May 2020. MMWR. 2020;69:930-32. (This is the Centers for Disease Control [CDC] weekly report called Morbidity and Mortality Weekly Report [MMWR])
40. World Health Organization. Interim Guidance report June 5, 2020. Advice on the use of masks in the context of COVID-19.

41. Isaacs D, Britton P, Howard-Jones A, et al. Do facemasks protect against COVID-19? J Paediatrics Child Health. 2020;56:976-77.
42. Leung NH, Chu DK, Shiu EY, et al. Respiratory virus shedding in exhaled breath and efficacy of face masks. Nature Medicine. 2020;26:676-80.
43. NY Times. Poor Americans hit hardest by job losses amid lockdowns, Fed says. https://www.nytimes.com/2020/05/14/business/economy/coronavirus-jobless-unemployment.html
44. CNN 4.3 million homeowners missed their mortgage payments last month (May 2020) https://www.cnn.com/2020/06/22/success/mortgage-payment-delinquencies-in-may-coronavirus/index.html
45. Koenig D. The 'quarantine 15': Weight gain during the COVID-19 pandemic. May 24, 2020. https://www.medicinenet.com/the_quarantine_15_weight_gain_during_covid-19-news.htm

Index

Printed in Great Britain
by Amazon

55018217R00098